DIET AND EXERCISE: SYNERGISM IN HEALTH MAINTENANCE

Editors

Philip L. White, ScD
and
Therese Mondeika, RD

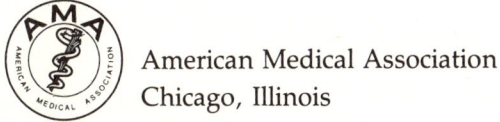

American Medical Association
Chicago, Illinois

Copyright © 1982 by the
American Medical Association
All rights reserved

Additional copies may be purchased from:
Order Department OP-163
American Medical Association
P.O. Box 10946
Chicago, Illinois 60610

ISBN: 0-89970-153-1

HCB:82-651:6M:12/82

SYMPOSIUM ON DIET AND EXERCISE: SYNERGISM IN HEALTH MAINTENANCE

November 3-4, 1981

Sponsored by the Department of Foods and Nutrition, Council on Scientific Affairs, and Council on Continuing Physician Education of the American Medical Association, and the Florida Medical Association

Program Committee:

Philip L. White, ScD, Chairman
Howard E. Bauman, PhD
E. R. Buskirk, PhD
C. Wayne Callaway, MD
Stephanie C. Crocco, PhD
Ray C. Frodey
J. Edward Hunter, PhD
Walter H. Meyer
Therese Mondeika, RD
Robert E. Olson, MD, PhD

TABLE OF CONTENTS

Contributors vii

Preface
   Philip L. White xi

Acknowledgments xiv

BALANCING THE EQUATION: PHYSICAL ACTIVITY AND NUTRITION

Importance of Physical Activity and Nutrition in Health Maintenance
   Robert E. Olson 3

Effects of Regular Physical Activity on the Physiology of Active and Sedentary Individuals
   E. R. Buskirk 15

Physical Activity and Dietary Intakes
   Nathan J. Smith 27

INTERRELATION OF PHYSICAL ACTIVITY AND NUTRITION

Interrelation of Physical Activity and Nutrition on Lipid Metabolism
   Peter D. Wood and William L. Haskell 39

Protein Metabolism and Exercise
   Robert A. Hoerr, Vernon R. Young, William J. Evans 49

Interrelation of Physical Activity and Nutrition on Blood Pressure/Circulation
   Richard M. Schieken 67

Some Influences on Lean Body Mass: Exercise, Androgens, Pregnancy, and Food
   Gilbert B. Forbes 75

Interrelation of Physical Activity and Nutrition on Obesity
   Per Björntorp 91

Interrelation of Physical Activity and Nutrition on Bone Mass
   G. Donald Whedon 99

RX: DIET AND ACTIVITY

Energy Imbalance and Hypertension Risk
   Ralph S. Paffenbarger 115

Physical Activity and Diet in the Treatment of Coronary Heart Disease
   Samuel M. Fox and James A. Metcalf 127

Exercise and Diet in the Therapy of Diabetes
  Neil B. Ruderman, Stephen H. Schneider, Louis Amoroso,
  Dieter Kramsch... 143

The Role of Diet and Activity in the Treatment of Osteoporosis
  Robert P. Heaney... 153

CONTRIBUTORS

Louis Amoroso, MD
Associate Professor of Clinical Medicine
Division of Endocrinology and Metabolism
New Jersey College of Medicine
Piscataway, NJ 08854

Per Björntorp, MD
Department of Medicine
Sahlgren's Hospital
Goteborg, Sweden

E. R. Buskirk, PhD
Director
Laboratory for Human Performance Research
The Pennsylvania State University
University Park, PA 16802

William J. Evans, PhD
Assistant Professor of Physiology
Department of Health Sciences
Boston University
Boston, MA 02215

Gilbert B. Forbes, MD
Professor of Pediatrics
Department of Pediatrics
The University of Rochester Medical Center
Rochester, NY 14642

Samuel M. Fox, III, MD
Professor of Medicine
Director, Preventive Cardiology Program
Georgetown University Hospital
Washington, DC 20007

William L. Haskell, PhD
Clinical Associate Professor of Medicine
Stanford Heart Disease Prevention Program
Stanford University Medical Center
Stanford, CA 94305

Robert P. Heaney, MD
Vice President for Health Sciences
Creighton University
Omaha, NE 68178

Robert A. Hoerr, MD
Assistant Director
Clinical Research Center
Massachusetts Institute of Technology
Cambridge, MA 02139

Dieter Kramsch, MD
Assistant Professor of Medicine
Assistant Professor of Biochemistry
Division of Diabetes and Metabolism
Departments of Physiology and Biochemistry
Boston University Medical Center
Boston, MA 02118

James A. Metcalf, PhD
Associate Professor of Health and Physical Education
George Mason University
Fairfax, VA 22030

Robert E. Olson, MD
Alice A. Doisy Professor and Chairman
Department of Biochemistry
St. Louis University School of Medicine
St. Louis, MO 63104

Ralph S. Paffenbarger, Jr., MD, DrPH
Professor of Epidemiology
Stanford University School of Medicine
Stanford, CA 94305

Neil B. Ruderman, MD, DPhil
Professor of Medicine and Physiology
Chief, Division of Diabetes and Metabolism
Boston University Medical Center
Boston, MA 02118

Richard M. Schieken, MD
Professor, Pediatric Cardiology
Department of Pediatrics
The University of Iowa Hospitals and Clinics
Iowa City, IA 52242

Stephen H. Schneider, MD
Assistant Professor of Medicine
Division of Endocrinology and Metabolism
New Jersey College of Medicine
Piscataway, NJ 08854

Nathan J. Smith, MD
Professor
Department of Pediatrics and Orthopedics
 (Sports Medicine)
University of Washington
School of Medicine
Seattle, WA 98195

G. Donald Whedon, MD
Senior Science Advisor
National Institute of Arthritis, Diabetes,
 and Digestive and Kidney Diseases
National Institutes of Health
Bethesda, MD 20205

Peter D. Wood, DSc
Adjunct Professor of Medicine
Deputy Director, Stanford Heart Disease
 Prevention Program
Stanford University Medical Center
Stanford, CA 94305

Vernon R. Young, PhD
Professor of Nutritional Biochemistry
Department of Nutrition and Food Science
 and Clinical Research Center
Massachusetts Institute of Technology
Cambridge, MA 02139

PREFACE

Exercise physiologists have always been convinced of the health benefits of appropriate exercise, but now they are involved with management of disease risks as well. To what degree does exercise influence the plasma lipoprotein concentrations? Is the exercised, conditioned obese individual at lower risk of developing cardiovascular problems or diabetes, hypertension or osteoporosis than the sedentary obese counterpart?

The AMA Council on Scientific Affairs considered these matters in its statement, *American Medical Association Concepts of Nutrition and Health (JAMA* 242:2335–2338, 1979):

"Many problems associated with the 'usual American diet' and 'American food habits' reflect abandonment of the dictum of *moderation*. Immoderate habits, namely, overeating, may exacerbate or contribute to the development of degenerative diseases. Contemporary concerns about diet and disease center on the kinds and amounts of fatty acids and carbohydrates in the diet, the amounts of sodium, plant fibers, cholesterol, alcohol, and total calories, and also the level of energy expenditure in physical activity.

A common denominator of the various dietary guidelines proposed to modify the risks of chronic and degenerative diseases is the emphasis on restraint or *moderation*. Few would argue against the concept of 'all things in moderation,' though many would say that it is paltry advice in an era unsurpassed in advances in biomedical research. In time, when our knowledge of the relationships, if any, of specific food components to the development of chronic diseases reaches maturity, it may be feasible to make more refined recommendations. Until then, *the AMA recommends that the American public give primary emphasis to the achievement and maintenance of the most desirable body weight and further recommends that this be accomplished through the combination of dietary control and exercise.*

This recommendation is considered the most appropriate for healthy people, but is also applicable to large numbers of Americans who are at greater risk for certain diseases and to those who must contend with specific dietary modifications instituted for the management of hypertension, diabetes, coronary heart disease, and other medical problems."

The emphasis of the Council statement was on diet and exercise to achieve and maintain the most desirable body weight. Perhaps it would have been more to the point to have stressed desirable body composition; a desirable body weight *per se* is not necessarily an appropriate benchmark of health. Enhancement of health and performance certainly is related to the relative proportion of lean body tissue, skeletal mass and energy stores and the use to which these body compartments are placed. More simply stated, the appropriate combination of diet and exercise should lead to a beneficial homeostatic set point appropriate for optimal health. If that be the case, there may be a synergistic effect between diet and exercise, ie, the working together in such fashion that the total effect is greater than the sum of the effects taken independently. For example, the object in weight reduction is to permit a transition from the physical and physiological conditions characteristic of obesity to those characteristic of leanness without incurring irreversible damage in the process. The combination of exercise and diet appears to be synergistic in the creation of an energy deficit. There also appears to be a synergistic effect on plasma lipoprotein concentrations, and perhaps on carbohydrate utilization in the non-insulin-dependent-diabetic state, somewhat characteristic of obesity.

We arrive, then, at the origin of the Symposium that spawned this book. The Food Industry Liaison Advisory Panel of the Department of Foods and Nutrition and the Department's Nutrition Advisory Group in clinical nutrition designed the program to examine the physiologic effects of moderate habitual physical activity and sound nutritional practices, independently and collectively. The effects were to be reviewed from the standpoints of health maintenance and treatment of certain of the major health problems in this country. The Symposium was designed to focus on the condition of chronic (regular) adaptation to exercise rather than on the acute "nonsteady" state of exercise or on the extremely vigorous activity of maximum performance. It was recognized that less information would be available on the effects of "moderate" regular exercise than on the effects of maximal physical performance. If there are optimum amounts of physical activity needed for measurable benefits, it was hoped that the Symposium could help to define those levels.

The program planners had envisioned the Gaussian Curve with inactivity at one extreme and sustained vigorous activity at the other. Within that range of physical activity the following questions were posed:

1. What are the "knowns" regarding the physical and physiological effects of diet and activity?
2. Is there reason to surmise that exercise superimposed on any variation of diet is beneficial?
3. Has the type of exercise (or diet) been identified?
4. Can the available data on the effects of exercise, diet, and exercise-diet support any specific recommendations for application in health maintenance and/or therapy?
5. What research priorities can be identified?

The book is organized to progress from the effects of exercise and the effects of diet on the whole body through their effects on metabolism, the circulatory system and bone mass. The last section reviews the influence of exercise and diet on the treatment of CHD, diabetes, hypertension, and osteoporosis. Following the general introductory chapter on the importance of both physical activity and nutrition in health maintenance, the chapters become quite specific. They lay the groundwork of the influences of diet and exercise on normal and abnormal physiology that leads into the chapters on exercise and diet in the prevention and treatment of disease. Three of the papers presented at the Symposium were not submitted for publication and are, therefore, not included in this book. Unless otherwise noted, each chapter considers the effects of diet and activity individually and combined, searching, as it were, for synergistic effects.

A clear message echoes throughout the book. The human body performs best when it is regularly stressed by appropriate physical exercise and is properly nourished. A number of physiological synergisms expressing the added benefits of nutrition and exercise have been identified. The maintenance of a healthful homeostasis (or the return to that state) usually involves a proper combination of diet and exercise. One can not substitute for the other.

Approaches to health and its maintenance should be positive and enjoyable. Whatever is required to achieve health and hold onto it must be sustainable throughout life. Motivation to commit oneself to a life of proper diet and exercise may require more information about mechanics than is currently available. In the final analysis, the search is for an understanding of the permissible physical and physiological latitudes that are commensurate with good health.

Philip L. White, ScD

ACKNOWLEDGMENTS

The generous financial support of the following organizations is deeply appreciated:

1. Best Foods, CPC International
2. Campbell Soup Company
3. The Coca-Cola Company
4. Dr. Pepper Company
5. Frito-Lay, Inc.
6. General Foods Corporation
7. General Mills, Inc.
8. Hershey Foods Corporation
9. Hoffman-La Roche Inc.
10. ITT Continental Baking Company Inc.
11. Kellogg Company
12. Kraft Inc.
13. Lever Brothers Company
14. Life Savers, Inc.
15. McCormick & Company, Inc.
16. Nabisco, Inc.
17. The Pillsbury Company
18. The Procter & Gamble Company
19. Quaker Oats Company
20. Ross Laboratories
21. Stouffer Foods Corporation
22. Weight Watchers International
23. Wm. Underwood Company

BALANCING THE EQUATION: PHYSICAL ACTIVITY AND NUTRITION

Moderator: Terence Kavanagh, MD, DPhysMed
Medical Director
Toronto Rehabilitation Centre
Toronto, Ontario

IMPORTANCE OF PHYSICAL ACTIVITY AND NUTRITION IN HEALTH MAINTENANCE

Robert E. Olson, MD, PhD*

Health is not just the absence of illness. The World Health Organization stated, "Health is a state of complete physical, mental and social well-being and not merely the absence of disease or infirmity".[1] The maintenance of health is as multidimensional as the causation of illness. It is futile to discuss health maintenance in terms of single factors. Good nutrition, physical fitness, proper genes, internal homeostasis, social adjustment, and personal happiness all contribute to good health. In most of us, health protection is quite secure and multiple attack is necessary to penetrate that armor.

Both health and illness are of multiple etiology. The agent of a disease is only one cause but it is an essential cause. The agents of health are biochemical and maintain the proper structure and function of all cells aided by multiple layers of enzymatic, immunochemical and structural defenses against noxious agents. These defenses neutralize many assaults by toxic agents. Multiple causation is thus universal in medicine for both health and disease.

Strategy in Public Health

In attacking a public health problem, effective intervention against disease depends on attacking the most vulnerable link in a chain of multiple causation. For example, during a cholera epidemic in London in 1849, John Snow concluded, on purely epidemiological grounds, that the Broad Street pump was the source of infection. By removing the handle of the pump, he was able to prevent the disease in that part of London. This attack on the environment was effective despite the lack of knowledge concerning the causative agent. Many years later, Phillips[2] discovered that the morbid pathophysiology of cholera depended on the depletion of intracellular fluid since cholera toxin reverses sodium transport in gastrointestinal cells. His strategy, therefore, was not to attack the organism, but to replace the fluids which were being lost through gastrointestinal secretions. A less successful strategy for control of coronary heart disease through dietary fat modification has had no effect on overall mortality in eight clinical trials.[3,4] It is likely that new strategies involving multiple intervention will be necessary to control the more complicated degenerative diseases.

---

*St. Louis University School of Medicine, St. Louis, Missouri.

In view of these complications, it is not useful for health professionals in one field to insist that their respective modality of prevention, even if demonstrated to be partially effective, is the best approach to the promotion of health and prevention of disease. In fact, I believe there is too much emphasis on diet at the present time and insufficient attention being given to other important factors in the prevention of disease, eg, immunization, promotion of physical fitness, avoidance of cigarette smoking and drug abuse, and risk factor assessment by health professionals.

To be successful, nutritional approaches must be multidimensional. In addition to supplying essential nutrients, macronutrient ratios must be adjusted to provide the best package for the delivery of calories to given individuals. There appears to be a wide variation in individual responses to various macronutrient intakes as measured by the preservation of homeostasis with respect to blood levels of glucose, amino acids, cholesterol, triglycerides and lipoproteins.

This book is devoted to diet and exercise and the conclusion is anticipated by the phrase in the title "synergism in health maintenance". Physical activity *and* nutrition are both very important for the maintenance of health. Perhaps more emphasis should now be put on stimulating physical activity in our population in order to redress a growing imbalance in public health education.

Recommended Dietary Allowances

The approximately 44 essential nutrients for adult human beings are presented in Table 1 in amounts recommended by the Food and Nutrition Board.[5] This is shown to remind us that the vocabulary required to communicate nutrition information in this form requires scientific training in chemistry. This is suitable for medical students and many health professionals but is not suitable for the average layman who is interested in obtaining these 44 chemicals in adequate amounts from foods. To this end, food groupings were used by the United States Department of Agriculture (USDA) as early as 1916 to teach the composition of the balanced diet.

The current USDA Daily Food Guide recommends a daily minimum intake of four servings of fruits and vegetables, four servings of cereals and grains, two servings of dairy products and two servings of the meat group which contains legumes as well as red meat, fish and fowl. A fifth group which includes fats, sweets, and alcohol is included in the Daily Food Guide. The amount of these foods to use, however, depends on the calorie requirements of the individual. Energy intake should be adjusted to maintain a desired body weight at a suitable level for physical activity. The vocabulary here involves foods and not nutrients. This message has been successfully communicated to many individuals and is the mainstay of nutrition education in the schools, colleges and in continuing education programs.

The Food and Nutrition Board was created by Franklin D. Roosevelt during World War II. The Board was charged with the responsibility of encouraging nutritional practices by the US population that would allow for maintenance and

Table 1. A Chemically Defined Adequate Daily Diet for a Sedentary 22 Year Old Adult Man

Name	Amount		Name	Amount		Name	Amount	
WATER	2500	ml	**CALORIES**			**BULK**		
			Glucose	600	g	Cellulose	20	g
MINERALS			Triolein	20	g			
Ammonium acetate	20.0	g				**VITAMINS**		
Calcium acid phosphate	3.0	g	**AMINO ACIDS**			Ascorbic Acid	60	mg
Sodium chloride	4.0	g	L-Leucine	2.2	g	Niacin	18	mg
Potassium chloride	4.0	g	L-Phenylalanine	1.9	g	Vitamin E	10	mg
Magnesium carbonate	1.0	g	L-Lysine	1.8	g	Pantothenate	7	mg
Zinc sulfate	40	mg	L-Valine	1.6	g	Pyridoxine	2.0	mg
Ferrous sulfate	25	mg	L-Isoleucine	1.3	g	Riboflavin	1.7	mg
Manganese sulfate	10	mg	L-Methionine	1.2	g	Thiamin	1.5	mg
Copper sulfate	7	mg	L-Threonine	1.3	g	Vitamin A	1.0	mg
Sodium fluoride	2	mg	L-Tryptophan	0.4	g	Folate	0.4	mg
Sodium molybdate	1	mg				Biotin	0.2	mg
Chromium sulfate	0.6	mg	**FATTY ACIDS**			Vitamin K	0.1	mg
Sodium selenate	0.5	mg	Trilinolein	10.0	g	Vitamin D	.01	mg
Potassium iodide	0.2	mg	Trilinolenin	1.0	g	Vitamin B_{12}	.003	mg

The above amounts of essential nutrients are based on the RDA for a 22 year old male weighing 70 kg (RDA NRC, 1980).[5] Included are nutrients which are known to be essential for man but for which an RDA has not yet been established. In these cases, the top value for the ranges recommended as "Estimated Safe and Adequate Daily Dietary Intakes of Selected Vitamins and Minerals" is used. Linolenate is now established as essential for man.[6] In addition, four additional minerals known to be required by animals,[7] should be added to purified diets for man. These are silicon (50 mg/day); vanadium (200 μg/day); nickel (50 μg/day); and tin (500 μg/day).

promotion of health. The first problem undertaken by the Board was the assembly of a data base which would enable it to make recommendations regarding amounts of essential nutrients that would assure adequate nutrition in the US population. Such allowances were calculated to exceed average nutritional requirements by a safety margin related to the statistical spread of requirements in a normal population.

If one studies the vitamin, mineral, amino acid and energy requirements of a respective group of healthy persons, one will obtain in each case a range of requirements which will approach a normal distribution curve. On the basis of a statistical analysis of such a curve, one can conclude that two standard deviations above the mean requirement will encompass 97.5% of the people at risk. Recommended Dietary Allowances (RDAs) are thus defined as levels of intake of essential nutrients, considered in the judgement of the Food and Nutrition Board, on the basis of available scientific knowledge, to be adequate to meet the known nutritional needs of practically all healthy people. The cutting point, therefore, is placed at the high end of the range of nutritional requirements and, by definition, is higher than the requirements of 97% of the population. This point is sometimes overlooked when RDAs are used for various purposes other than those for which it was intended, namely, planning adequate diets for populations.

The Food and Nutrition Board bases its recommendations on a large body of data. These data are derived from epidemiologic studies; studies of the clinical management of overt deficiency diseases; clinical investigations in which the diet is altered to a nutritional level below and then above the requirement of the individual subject, using appropriate biochemical indicators; clinical trials in which supplementation or fortification is used to control nutritional disease in populations; and, finally, studies in appropriate animal models.

The Food and Nutrition Board has revised the RDAs nine times since 1943. The ninth edition was published in 1980.[5] The increase in the number of nutrients for which RDAs have been established over four decades (8 in 1943 and 18 in 1980) illustrates the evolution of knowledge in the field. This evolution and refinement of the RDAs will continue as additional data become available. Refinement of information about the optimum intake of macronutrients for health promotion will also occur as the Food and Nutrition Board develops the second edition of "Toward Healthful Diets".[8] This changing information must be communicated to the public *in toto* in order that the nutritional component in any health maintenance program remains current.

One of the unfortunate developments occurring in the United States is the increasing sedentary character of our population. The associated reduced food intake, according to the recent USDA survey of household food-consumption,[9] supplies an average of only 1500 kcal/day for middle-aged women and 2200 kcal/day for middle-aged men. This level of energy exchange, which is near basal rates, has so reduced food intake that the RDAs for some micronutrients are not attainable with ordinary food selection. This has led to cries for food fortification by some. Conversely, my view is to recommend a 10% increase in physical activity. The corresponding increase in food intake would be sufficient to provide adequate intakes of all of the essential nutrients from ordinary foods.

Physical Activity

Physical activity is very important for health. Its importance has been demonstrated in studies covering both extremes—from the immobilized, chronically ill person who is unable to walk to the olympic class athlete who is in a state of peak physical fitness. It is clear from clinical experience and investigation that immobilization and bed rest diminish physical fitness. There is a reduction in exercise tolerance, an increased heart rate on exertion, loss of calcium and phosphorus from bones, and potassium from muscles. Various degrees of physical fitness result from conditioning at all levels of activity, from the very minimum physical capacity of the invalid to the high levels of work performance of the professional athlete. As in most dynamic states, one is never stationary but is either gaining or losing fitness. Personal experience teaches us that if one suddenly curtails a physical fitness program that involves jogging, running, calisthenics or aerobic dancing, one drifts toward inactivity with a corresponding loss of fitness. Physical activity is thus a prime requirement for health promotion.

Physical Activity and Disease Prevention

How much physical activity is enough? Clement Atlee said he owed his long life to resisting all forms of exercise. On the other hand, studies have shown that a level of exercise equivalent to an expenditure of 2000 kcal/week above the ordinary level, ie, 2500 kcal/day in men, will not only maintain fitness but decrease the risk of coronary heart disease (CHD) and stroke.[10-12] This represents a mere 11% increase over "ordinary activity".

Many geographic studies have suggested that dietary fat, particularly saturated fat, is an important risk factor for hypercholesterolemia and CHD. This epidemiologic evidence has been contradicted by findings in the Masai in Tanzania in whom a high intake of milk and blood fat was associated with low cholesterol levels and a low incidence of CHD.[13] This led some to believe that certain peoples, like the Japanese and possibly Masai, are innately less liable to develop CHD than most Caucasians. The Japanese, however, who migrated to the United States have higher serum cholesterol levels and more atherosclerotic heart disease than do their compatriots in Japan.[14]

The Ireland-Boston Heart study, sometimes known as the Irish Brothers Study,[15] was designed to get around this particular difficulty by eliminating racial and, to some extent, broad hereditary differences while at the same time ensuring considerable environmental variation by taking for the main cohort, 1,154 Irish brothers who lived several thousand miles apart. Matched within ten years of each others age, 579 were living in Boston and 575 were living in Ireland. In addition, there were 376 first generation Irish-Americans born of immigrants (in the age range of 20–60 years) who were studied and some other smaller contrast groups. A total of 1,194 men were studied over a period of four years from 1960–1964. As shown in Table 2, the dietary intakes for fat, saturated fat and cholesterol were higher in the brothers living in Ireland than those living in Boston; however, serum cholesterol levels were similar, tricep skin folds were thinner and body weights lower in the former group. Blood pressure levels and smoking habits were similar in both groups, although more EKG abnormalities were found in the Boston Irish.

Although overall mortality rates per 100,000 male population in the United States and Ireland in 1950 were similar at age 55-64, mortality rates from CHD averaged 300 more per 100,000 in the United States than in Ireland. (Table 3)

Table 2. Ireland-Boston Heart Study (1970)*

Characteristic	First Generation (n = 376)	Boston Brothers (n = 579)	Irish Brothers (n = 575)
DIET			
Calories	2984 ± 880**	3075 ± 771	3768 ± 1132
Fat (g)	131 ± 46	135 ± 43	159 ± 55
P/S ratio	0.21 ± 0.13	0.16 ± 0.09	0.12 ± 0.04
Cholesterol (mg)	696 ± 261	844 ± 312	894 ± 345
Alcohol (g)	34 ± 36	36 ± 37	16 ± 22
BLOOD PRESSURE			
Systolic (mm Hg)	135 ± 21	137 ± 21	135 ± 19
Diastolic (mm Hg)	85 ± 12	86 ± 13	83 ± 11
SERUM CHOLESTEROL			
mg/dl	215 ± 42	219 ± 39	213 ± 44
BODY WEIGHT (lbs)	176 ± 26	172 ± 23	162 ± 26
TRICEPS SKIN-FOLD (mm)	13 ± 7	10 ± 4	7 ± 4

*Adapted Brown J, et al[15]
**Variance is given as standard deviation

Table 3. Mortality Rates per 100,000 males population (1950)

Age Range	All causes		Classification 420–422*	
	U.S.	Ireland	U.S.	Ireland
45–54	1067	922	348	199
55–64	2046	2044	896	596

*Classification 420–422 = arteriosclerotic and myocardial heart disease. Reproduced with permission from *World Rev Nutr Diet.*[15] (Courtesy of Karger, Basel))

The brothers in Ireland ate more food yet weighed less than their brothers in Boston. Contemporary autopsies also showed much earlier serious atheromatosis of aorta and coronary arteries in the Boston subjects as compared with those living in Ireland. The Irish brothers are more active physically than their brothers in Boston and this difference correlates with a change in the mortality rate from atherosclerotic heart disease. Increased physical activity, apart from diet and serum cholesterol levels, appears to reduce the risk of CHD.

In the United States, Krauss et al[16] reported that the degree of exercise in previously healthy sedentary men age 30 to 55, correlated with the rise in HDL-cholesterol and a fall in LDL-cholesterol. The extent of exercise also correlated with loss of body fat. It was concluded that exercise promotes metabolic processes that modulate coronary disease risk. The Food and Nutrition Board in its report "Toward Healthful Diets",[8] recommended increased physical activity as well as a diet composed of a variety of foods chosen from the USDA's Daily Food Guide. The Board believed that these two recommendations were the best guidelines for disease prevention and health promotion.

Spontaneous Changes In Coronary Heart Disease

Although coronary heart disease (CHD) was first recognized as a clinical entity by Herrick in 1912, the lesions of the disease have been seen by pathologists for centuries. Epidemiologists have been captivated by the spotaneous changes in mortality rates from CHD. In the United States, there was a remarkable increase in mortality rates from coronary disease between 1912 and 1963, which led to the view that CHD was an uncontrolled epidemic in this country. Unexpectedly, however, the mortality rate from CHD in the United States has been decreasing at the rate of 1% to 2% per year since 1963 for obscure reasons which are being studied in this country and elsewhere.

Several countries are currently experiencing a decrease in death rate from CHD. In the United States, the decrease of 28 per 100,000 in four years is greater than elsewhere, as shown in Table 4, but an equal number of countries are showing an increase of even greater magnitude. The northern European countries of Germany, Sweden, Norway, England, Denmark, Northern Ireland and Scotland experienced increased mortality of from 9 to 43 per 100,000 between 1969 and 1973. The reasons for this, even in the Scandinavian countries which have had recommendations from their governments for eight years which parallel the "Dietary Goals for the U.S.", are far from clear.[17]

The US Department of Health, Education and Welfare held a conference in May 1979, to study the decline in CHD mortality in the United States.[18] It reached the following conclusions: 1) the decrease in CHD mortality is real and not the result of artifacts or changes in death certificate coding, 2) both primary prevention through changes in risk factors and fundamental clinical research, leading to better care, probably have contributed to, but do not fully explain, the decline, and 3) a precise quantification of the causes requires further study, especially those designed to document whether the frequency of non-fatal coronary events is changing.

Since 1968, the downward trend in CHD mortality has been seen in men and women, whites and blacks, and for all adult ages. The overall rate of decline has been greatest among black women.

Improved medical care such as specialized hospital procedures for monitoring, preventing and treating cardiac arrhythmias has become the standard aspect of the treatment of individuals with acute myocardial infarction. The

Table 4. Trend in the Death Rate for Coronary Heart Disease Selected Countries, 1969–73 Males Age 45–54 Years

Country	Difference in Death Rate	Rate per 100,000 Population	
		1969	1973
United States	−28.3	341.2	312.9
Canada	−24.6	273.1	248.5
Australia	−18.4	314.7	296.3
Finland	−17.1	427.3	410.2
Israel	−15.1	203.2	188.1
Japan	− 3.7	34.4	30.7
Austria	− 0.4	146.7	146.3
Italy	+ 0.6	112.9	113.5
Netherlands	+ 2.5	188.8	191.3
Switzerland	+ 4.1	103.4	107.5
Germany, F.R.	+ 9.3	146.4	155.7
Hungary	+21.5	142.8	164.3
Sweden	+30.1	126.0	156.1
Norway	+31.1	191.5	222.6
England and Wales	+31.6	254.9	286.5
Denmark	+31.9	159.5	191.4
Northern Ireland	+43.2	318.9	362.1
Scotland	+43.5	329.2	372.7

The reprint of 1977 Working Group to review Arteriosclerosis: From U.S. DHEW Publication (NIH) 78-1526. 1971 Report by NHLBI Task Force on Atherosclerosis.

reported mortality occurring from acute CHD treated in hospitals fell from 30% to 20% in the past decade. It must be realized, however, that 70% of CHD deaths occur out of a hospital. There have been improvements in both medical and surgical care of CHD. Coronary bypass surgery has increased exponentially, but its widespread use is recent and could not have affected mortality rates in the 1960s.

CHD mortality is decreasing at a faster rate than general mortality which is also falling. Since 1900, the crude death rate in the United States has fallen from 17 deaths to less than 9 per 1000.[19] The decrease is characteristic of all age groups. Many causes of death (except lung cancer, chronic lung disease and suicide-homicide) are falling at the same rate as CHD. Jones[20] has suggested that this positive force for health is a more vigorous and illness-free childhood.

Since the decline is distributed throughout all age groups, it is probably due more to a change in risk factors than in medical care. It should be appreciated, however, that 50% of the risk from CHD is not explained by the presently known risk factors which include maleness, family history, hypertension, hypercholesterolemia, obesity, diabetes, and cigarette smoking. Although the percentage of smokers and the amount of tar and nicotine in cigarettes have dropped in this country since the release of the first Surgeon General's report in 1964,[21] the frequency of individuals smoking two or more packs of cigarettes per day has not changed, according to at least one survey. In addition, women, who have enjoyed the greatest decline in mortality, have inconsistently changed their smoking habits. Consumption of cigarettes did increase during the post-World War I era, which may have affected the subsequent increase in coronary heart disease deaths, and it is now estimated that the average fall in CHD mortality is about 20%. There is no convincing temporal relationship between smoking and CHD mortality as exists for smoking and lung cancer.

There is substantial evidence that the awareness and effective treatment of hypertension have increased dramatically over the last decade. Therapy for hypertension is instituted only in those with blood pressures in the upper 5% or 10% of the population distribution, so that it is not unexpected that the mean blood pressure level for the population has not changed substantially. Improved therapy for hypertension is an appealing explanation of some of the decline in mortality, since there has been a greater drop in mortality in women, especially black women. It is this group which, presumably, has taken greatest advantage of treatment for hypertension. The recent National Heart, Lung, and Blood Institute (NHLBI) study of the effects of stepped drug treatment of hypertension has demonstrated a 17% reduction in five-year mortality.[22] On the other hand, mortality from hypertensive heart disease and stroke began to decline some years before effective medical therapy for hypertension was available and during a time when CHD mortality was increasing.

There have been nutritional changes over recent years associated with decreases in consumption of eggs and butter and increases in intake of polyunsaturated fats, but these changes do not bear an appropriate temporal relationship to the changes in incidence of CHD. Total fat intake has increased due to increased consumption of vegetable oils. The increasing frequency of obesity in certain segments of the population suggests excess calorie consumption over energy expended. The net effect on blood cholesterol levels can not be determined accurately but it appears that there may have been an overall reduction in blood cholesterol levels of 3% to 5% over the last ten years.

If improved therapy for hypertension and reduced smoking are considered along with the small reduction in serum cholesterol, some of the decline in CHD mortality can be explained. Cornfield[23] warned against applying natural risk factor prediction to changes in these risk factors due to multiple interventions. He concluded that there was no available mathematical model which had been validated for that purpose. The failure of numerous diet and drug trials, which have lowered serum cholesterol values 6% to 16% over a four year period, to alter mortality illustrates the difficulties of predicting results from data available for the whole US population. Various well-planned clinical trials of such interventions are underway and these should provide some answers to these questions.

Exercise and, in particular, jogging have increased in frequency in the United States, but this trend has been a recent development and has involved only certain groups. Its effect on a decline in mortality beginning in the mid-1960s must be minimal, although it is possible that its true effect will be determined in the future.

The attempt in the United States to impose numerous dietary guidelines designed to further reduce the incidence and mortality rates for CHD may be unnecessary. The spectacular decline in CHD mortality is occurring in a country with minimal change in dietary patterns, except for a general reduction in energy expenditure. The idea that there is consensus among health professionals in the United States that dietary patterns need to be changed because DHEW and USDA have published non-quantitative guidelines which mimic in general the "Dietary Goals of the U.S." of the McGovern committee is misleading.[24]

It is tempting to believe that a combination of small changes in a number of environmental factors such as diet, smoking, physical exercise, and drugs for the treatment of hypertension may be responsible for the decrease in CHD mortality in the United States and elsewhere. Certainly, diet is not responsible for much of the change. Other explanations are possible and the present controversy regarding the cause and effect relationship between environmental factors and CHD rates only emphasizes the need for more research into causation and development of new strategies for prevention of CHD.

Summary

Good nutrition and physical activity are both important determinants of health. The selection of a nourishing diet from the Daily Food Guide, using as wide a variety of foods as possible in amounts necessary to achieve an appropriate weight for height, is the best nutritional advice available for healthy people. Furthermore, increasing physical activity by 10% in the US population will improve physical fitness, increase micronutrient intake by permitting a corresponding increase in food intake, and may be an important factor in the prevention of coronary heart disease and stroke.

References

1. *World Health Organization Chronicle* 1:(13), 29–42, 1947.
2. Phillips RA: Water and electrolyte losses in cholera. *Fed Proc* 23:705–712, 1964.
3. Ahrens EH: The management of hyperlipidemias. Whether rather than how? *Ann Int Med* 85:87–93, 1976.
4. Olson RE: Obstacles to success in nutrition intervention programs: Inappropriate priorities, in Selvey N, White PL (eds): *Nutrition in the 1980s, Constraints on our Knowledge*. New York, AR Liss, 1981, pp 523–537.
5. Food and Nutrition Board: *Recommended Dietary Allowances*. National Academy of Sciences, National Research Council, Ninth Edition, Washington, DC, 1980.
6. Holman RT, Johnson SB, Hatch TF: Linolenic acid deficiency in man. *Nutr Rev* 40:144–147, 1982.
7. Mertz W: The essential trace elements. *Science* 213:1332–1338, 1981.
8. Food and Nutrition Board: *Toward Healthful Diets*. National Academy of Sciences, National Research Council, Washington, DC, 1980.
9. Peterkin BP: Nationwide food consumption survey, in Selvey N, White PL (eds): *Nutrition in the 1980s, Constraints on our Knowledge*. New York, AR Liss, 1981, pp 59–70.
10. Paffenbarger RS, Laughlin ME, Gima AS, et al: Work activity of longshoremen as related to death from coronary heart disease and stroke. *N Eng J Med* 282:1109–1114, 1970.
11. Paffenbarger RS, Wing AL, Hyde RT: Physical activity as an index of heart attack risk in college alumni. *Am J Epidemiol* 108:161–175, 1978.
12. Morris JN, Pollard R, Everett MG, et al: Vigorous exercise in leisure-time; protection against coronary heart disease. *Lancet* II:1207–1210, 1980.
13. Mann GV, Shaffer RD, Anderson RS, et al: Cardiovascular disease in the Masai. *J Atherosclerosis Research* 4:289–294, 1964.
14. Gordon T: Mortality experience among the Japanese in the United States, Hawaii and Japan. *Public Health Rep* 72:543–551, 1957.
15. Brown J, Bourke GJ, Gearty GF, et al: Nutritional and epidemiologic factors related to heart disease. *World Rev Nutr Diet* 12:1–42, 1970.
16. Krauss RM, Lindgren FT, Word PD, et al: Coordinate changes in serum lipoprotein subclasses during exercise conditioning. *Arteriosclerosis* 1:383A, 1981.
17. Molitor GTT, Sweden A: Bellwether of future policy trends, in Chou M, Harmon DP (eds): *Critical Food Issues of the Eighties*, New York, Pergamon Press, 1979, pp 66–93.
18. Havlik R, Reinleib M (eds): *Proceedings of the Conference on the Decline in Coronary Heart Disease Mortality*. DHEW, Public Health Service, NIH 79–1610, May, 1979.
19. *Healthy People, The Surgeon General's Report on Health Promotion and Disease Prevention*. DHEW, Public Health Service 79–55071, July, 1979.

20. Jones HB: A special consideration of the aging process, disease, and life expectancy. *Adv Biol Med Phys* 4:281–333, 1956.

21. Advisory Committee to the Surgeon General: *Smoking and health.* US Department of Health, Education & Welfare, PHS Publication No. 1103, 1964.

22. National Heart, Lung and Blood Institute: Five year findings of the hypertension detection and follow-up program. I. Reduction in mortality of persons with high blood pressure, including mild hypertension. *JAMA* 242:2562–2577, 1979.

23. Cornfield J. Joint dependence of risk of coronary heart disease on serum cholesterol and systolic blood pressure: a discriminant function analysis. *Fed Proc* 21 (suppl 2):58–61, 1962.

24. Olson RE: Integrating nutrition into medical and public health programs. *Food Technology* 34:58–61, 1980.

EFFECTS OF REGULAR PHYSICAL ACTIVITY ON THE PHYSIOLOGY OF ACTIVE AND SEDENTARY INDIVIDUALS

E. R. Buskirk, PhD*

Introduction

In discussing the physiological effects of regular exercise, with emphasis on nutritional aspects, it is important to identify certain concepts and provide definitions. The functional changes that occur in a progressive fashion with regular exercise are frequently referred to as responses, but perhaps the term should be reserved for those sudden and temporary alterations that result from participation in a single bout of exercise. The persistent changes in function and structure that accompany regular exercise yield what have been termed physical conditioning or training effects. Thus, adaptation is involved and, with repeated bouts of exercise, the conditioned body responds somewhat differently to additional exercise of the same type. The physiological strain associated with exercise is reduced. In a glossary of terms recommended for thermal physiology, adaptation was defined as a change which reduces the physiological strain produced by a stressful component of the total environment.[1]

Perhaps a differentiation should also be made between the term "physical conditioning" and the word "training." The latter term has been used extensively by physiologists, nutritionists and other scientists to describe changes related to a regimen of regular exercise, but "training" to coaches and others involved with athletes means preparation for competition. Improvement of athletic performance is the goal. A major component in improvement is the acquisition and development of specific athletic skills. In contrast, physical conditioning relates to the changes associated with the reduction in physiological strain brought about by regular exercise and it is this aspect which will be considered in this paper.

It should be borne in mind that adaptation takes time, involves genetic as well as environmental components, and is responsive to the type, frequency, intensity and duration of exercise. Adaptation is modified by factors which include age, maturation, sex, body build and body composition, among others. Adaptation brought about by physical conditioning may be viewed as an expected and useful biological phenomenon.

---

*The Pennsylvania State University, University Park, Pennsylvania.

Hettinger[2] stated the following principles for optimal adaptation:
1) an intensity-duration threshold must be exceeded to achieve an optimal rate of response
2) near continuous (ie, regular) exposure facilitates adaptation, and
3) intermission allows some deadaptation to occur that may be physiologically beneficial.

These principles were based on studies conducted by Hettinger and his colleagues on strength development and appear to apply to adaptations of most physiological systems.

The concept of negative feedback is important to keep in mind when considering adaptation to exercise; an example of negative feedback is body temperature regulation. There is an increase in deep body temperature during exercise. The increase is brought about by increased heat production in working muscle and is followed by sweating and increased blood flow to the skin. Heat loss is increased with evaporation of the sweat, as convective heat transfer occurs when the air moves past the skin. The result is that deep body temperature achieves a somewhat lower value than would have been the case had the heat loss mechanism not been activated. Thus, a relative thermal homeostasis is brought about through negative feedback. This feedback process tends to be modified so as to reduce physiological strain with adaptation to regular exercise.[3]

When one deals with exercise, concepts such as force, work, and power are involved, and the various types of muscle contraction—dynamic, isotonic, isometric, eccentric, concentric and isokinetic—must be considered. The words "work" and "exercise" are not synonymous, for work = force × distance. When a skeletal muscle is stimulated, it develops force by attempting to shorten itself along its longitudinal axis. The result will, in most cases, be a generation of torque through operation of this force upon one skeletal part, thereby tending to cause it to rotate around another. If skeletal movement is involved, muscle contraction is said to be dynamic, but requires further characterization as either concentric or eccentric. If this *attempt* at shortening is succesful, the contraction is termed concentric and involves the muscle's performance of work as defined above, ie, the acceleration of some mass or movement of an additional resisting component through a distance. If in spite of a muscle's attempt at shortening, it is in fact *lengthened*, the contraction is in this case termed eccentric, and work has been performed *upon* the muscle. Isometric muscle contraction or exercise, on the other hand, is not associated with either shortening or lengthening; only force (or torque) has been developed, with no work performed at all. Often, there is interest in the time required to perform physical work, in which case the concept of power is involved, ie, power = work × time $^{-1}$. The units of measurement used to describe work include newton-meters, kilocalories, joules, kilogram-meters and foot-pounds; units of power include Watts, kcal·t^{-1} and joules·t^{-1}. The terms are well clarified by Knuttgen, who offers several suggestions to investigators concerning their use.[4]

General Considerations

The factors that operate in a diverse population to modify physiological effects of regular exercise on nutrient requirements include the stage of growth, development and maturation; age; sex; physical condition; the climate or environment in which the exercise is regularly performed; disability or disease; and pregnancy and lactation. Most of these factors are considered in the *1980 Recommended Dietary Allowances*[5] and will not be covered here.

Regular exercise may not be enjoyable for all; however, in order to maintain physiological changes brought about by initial adherence to a regular exercise program, one has to exercise regularly. There are no shortcuts to the "overload" principles (ie, with muscles contracting under greater than normal loads) that are known at the present time. Thus, the regular exerciser must employ some motivational device; for some, it might be the enjoyment derived from regular exercise whereas the search for health benefits or the concept of "wellness" may suffice for others. Continued competition with one's self or others may also provide the necessary motivation.

Despite the increased interest in activities such as tennis, racketball, golf and jogging, walking remains the most popular form of exercise. Transporting one's body mass in walking provides a considerable metabolic stimulus. Depending on body weight, the extra calories expended per mile (assuming walking speeds of 3 to 4 mph) would range from about 50 to 100 kcal, the important factor being how far, not how fast, one walks. Jogging and running at slow speeds require more energy per mile than walking, but not all people feel comfortable when jogging or running. The physiological impact of walking on a regular basis remains significant.

Table 1. Classification of Physical Effort

Classification	$\dot{V}_E$	$\dot{V}_{O_2}$	MR or Mets	HR
Very light	<10	<0.5	<2.5	<80
Light	10–20	0.5–1.0	2.5–5.0	80–100
Moderate	20–35	1.0–1.5	5.0–7.5	100–120
Heavy	35–50	1.5–2.0	7.5–10.0	120–140
Very heavy	50–65	2.0–2.5	10.0–12.5	140–160
Unduly heavy	65–85	2.5–3.0	12.5–15.0	160–180
Exhausting	≥85	≥3.0	≥15.0	≥180

Abbreviations: $\dot{V}_E$, ventilation volume (liter·min^{-1}); $\dot{V}_{O_2}$, oxygen consumption (liter·min^{-1}); MR, caloric expenditure (kcal·min^{-1}); HR, heart rate (beats·min^{-1}).
The values listed apply to both steady-state work and peak effort for 70 kg man.

Adapted from Buskirk[6]

The diversity of exercise undertaken by different people is enormous; therefore, the physiological effects identifiable with regular exercise are, in many instances, task specific. Of necessity, investigators have classified physical effort according to common physiological variables such as heart rate, oxygen consumption and ventilation volume. A classification system of this type appears in Table 1.[6] Metabolic rate (MR) is expressed in $kcal \cdot min^{-1}$ and the values are roughly equivalent to Mets where 1 Met = 1.1 times the basal metabolic rate or approximately 3.5 ml $O_2 \cdot kg^1 \cdot min^{-1}$. The major deficiency of such a simple classification is that body mass, physical fitness, age, and sex are not taken into account.[7] Despite these shortcomings, it is a useful tool.

Metabolic Substrates

Although skeletal muscle constitutes about 40% of the body weight and has a low metabolic rate, its resting oxygen uptake corresponds to about 40% of body oxygen uptake. In contrast to many other tissues, it can increase metabolic turnover considerably, perhaps up to 50-fold. The muscles in individuals who are physically well-conditioned may have even higher turnovers. The energy reserves available in the body are set forth in Table 2. Lipid is the major reserve and is stored in adipose tissue while protein constitutes the next largest reserve and is stored in skeletal muscle. Although the carbohydrate reserves are relatively small, they are important in exercise metabolism.

Table 2. Estimates of the Major Energy Reserves of a Normal, Well-nourished 80 Kilogram Man

Tissue	Weight (kg)	Fuel	Amount (kg)	kcal
Adipose tissue	15	Triglyceride	14	135,000
Skeletal muscle	30	Triglyceride Protein Glycogen	0.3 6 0.4–0.6	2,500 24,500 1600–2500
Liver	1.8	Glycogen	0.09	360
Blood	6 liters	Glucose Triglyceride FFA	0.006 0.003 0.0004	24 30 4
			Approximate Total	164,400

If his daily energy expenditure is about 3,000 $kcal \cdot d^{-1}$, then the 80 kg man has a kcal turnover per day of about 1.8% of his kcal content.

From Gollnick (Personal Communication, October 1979)

During exercise, both carbohydrates and fat contribute significantly to the energy supply necessary to support muscular contraction and body movement. The proportions in the metabolic mixture are affected by both the intensity and the duration of exercise. During mild exercise, the proportion of carbohydrate and fat utilized is roughly equivalent to that of resting muscle. As the intensity of exercise increases, the proportion of carbohydrate utilization increases. When one nears the level of maximum exercise, much of the energy is derived from carbohydrate utilization with depletion of both liver and muscle glycogen reserves.[8,9]

Participation in regular exercise alters the rate of relative utilization of carbohydrate and fat during exercise. It has been demonstrated that rats adapted to exercise have an enhanced capability of utilizing fatty acids and ketones during submaximal exercise.[10,11] For example, palmitate oxidation was doubled in the leg muscles of rats who exercised regularly; presumably man responds in a similar fashion.[12] The increased utilization of fatty acids spares glucose utilization. Regular exercise appears to increase mobilization of fatty acids from lipid stored in adipose tissue and the elevated fatty acid (FFA) concentrations in blood apparently drive FFA oxidation. Lipoprotein lipase activity in both skeletal muscle and adipose tissue is relatively high in long distance runners.[13] Facilitation of fatty acid delivery from adipose tissue may well be accomplished by a relatively greater blood perfusion of both adipose tissue and skeletal muscle. Evidence to support such a concept, however, is not readily available other than the observation that an increased number of identifiable capillaries per skeletal muscle fiber may result from participation in regular exercise. For example, Ingjer and Brodal[14] found that the capillary per fiber ratio increased with increasing fiber diameter and mitochondrial content.

Physiological Effects

Astrand and Rodahl[15] summarized many of the physiological effects of regular exercise. Those significant effects that are directly or indirectly connected with nutrition appear in the following edited list:

Increases:
Strength of bones, ligaments and muscles
Muscle mass and body density
Articular cartilage thickness
Skeletal muscle ATP, CrP, K^+ and myoglobin
Skeletal muscle oxidative enzyme content and mitochondria
Skeletal muscle arterial collaterals and capillary density
Heart volume and weight
Blood volume and total circulating hemoglobin
Cardiac stroke volume
Maximal $C(a-v)O_2$
Maximal blood lactate concentration

Maximal pulmonary ventilation
Maximal respiratory work
Maximal oxygen diffusing capacity
Maximal exercise capacity as measured by the maximal oxygen intake, exercise time, and distance

Decreases:
Heart rate at rest and during submaximal exercise
Blood lactate concentration during submaximal exercise
Pulmonary ventilation during submaximal work
Respiratory quotient during submaximal work
Serum triglyceride concentration
Body fatness

On the basis of more recent evidence, the following effects might be added:

Increases:
Bone density
Myocardial contractility
Serum high density lipoprotein concentration
Anaerobic threshold
Plasma insulin concentration with submaximal exercise
Red blood cell and skeletal muscle receptor sites for some hormones

Decreases:
Serum low density lipoprotein concentration
Systolic blood pressure
Core temperature threshold for initiation of sweating
Sweat sodium and chloride content
Plasma epinephrine and norepinephrine with submaximal exercise
Plasma glucagon and growth hormone concentrations with submaximal exercise
Relative hemoconcentration with submaximal exercise in the heat

Increased vagal activity is presumably responsible for the decrease in resting heart rate brought about by regular exercise, but the mechanism is unknown.[16] Although the relationship between cardiac output and oxygen consumption is similar before and after engaging in a regimen of regular exercise, the stroke volume is greater and the heart rate less at each submaximal exercise intensity. Maximal heart rate remains unchanged, but maximal stroke volume is increased so that maximal cardiac output is increased. Genetic endowment also plays a role; the gifted runner undoubtedly has a larger stroke volume, total amount of hemoglobin and blood volume (see Table 3), and hence, a greater oxygen transport capability than can be brought about by regular running in those less well-endowed.[17]

Hepatic blood flow was found to be inversely proportional to the intensity of exercise whether exercise was performed under comfortable environmental

Table 3. Average Cardiovascular Values for Sedentary and Well-conditioned Men

	Heart wt. g / Body wt. kg	Heart Volume[1] (ml)	Blood Volume (liters)	Total Hemoglobin (g)
Sedentary men	5.8	769	5.3	805
Well-conditioned men	6.5	986	7.5	1130
Δ	+0.7	+217	+2.2	+325

[1]Resting, presystolic

(as summarized by Grande & Taylor[17])

conditions or in a hot air environment.[18] There was, however, a greater reduction under heat stress. Since the reduction in splanchnic blood flow appears to follow a straight line and negative slope relationship to relative exercise intensity (expressed as %$\dot{V}o_2$ max), improvement in aerobic capacity ($\dot{V}o_2$ max) with regular exercise would facilitate relatively greater splanchnic blood flows at submaximal exercise intensities. Exhausting exercise performance may well be compromised in a hot environment if hepatic blood flow is sufficiently reduced so that insufficient glucose is made available. Presumably, increased circulation through both the working muscle and the skin accounts for the reduction in splanchnic blood flow, including that which occurs through the kidney.

The relationship between the rate of sweating and deep body or core temperature is altered by a regimen of physical conditioning. Because the rate is controlled in part from temperature-sensitive areas in the hypothalamus, initiation of sweating at a lower core temperature is a useful adaptive feature. Evaporative cooling is initiated earlier and is maintained at higher rates following a regimen of regular exercise.[19] Neither the type nor intensity of exercise (positive compared to negative work) provided measurable exceptions to the modification of the regulation.[20] The capability for dissipating a larger thermal load during exercise via evaporative heat loss should provide the well-conditioned individual who is acclimated to heat with both a greater exercise capacity under warm or hot conditions and relatively lower peripheral circulatory demands during submaximal exercise. In the latter situation, deep body temperature would also be lower and tissue metabolic effects associated with the Q_{10} (ie, the change in metabolic turnover per 10°C change in temperature) temperature relationships would be reduced.

Regular exercise affects the balance between sympathetic and parasympathetic activities. Epinephrine and norepinephrine are normally released during exercise and plasma concentrations are proportional to exercise intensity. The increment is reduced following a regimen of regular exercise.[21] Plasma insulin concentrations tend to be relatively higher and glucagon lower with regular exercise.[22,23] Growth hormone in plasma may also increase,[21] as may thyroid hormone turnover.[24] The importance of these hormonal changes relative to metabolic substrate utilization and energy turnover remains to be resolved. Astrand and Rodahl[15] note ". . . many of the adaptations on a cellular level triggered by training are unique for the trained muscles, but are not found in 'idle' muscles which must be subjected to the same changes in hormone levels." Certainly, nutritional requirements are modified; the type and extent of the modification has yet to be resolved.

Knuttgen (personal communication, April 1981) has constructed a hypothetical example of what might happen to several physiological variables during regular aerobic exercise of two to three months and two to three years duration at an intensity of about 70% of the subject's aerobic capacity (see Table 4). He emphasizes that the power output is an important variable in any exercise prescription so that frequency, duration, type of exercise and intensity all play important roles.

The respective percentage changes depicted in Table 4 may be too great, particularly for variables such as the maximal oxygen intake and cardiac output

Table 4. Some Possible Physiological Effects of Regular Exercise for Several Months or Years in Subjects of Different Ages (18 years or 38 years). Estimated Percentage Increase

Variable	2 to 3 months		2 to 3 years	
	18 y	38 y	18 y	38 y
$\dot{V}O_2$ max (ml·kg^{-1}·min^{-1})	20	15	50	30
$\dot{Q}_{CO}$ (L·min^{-1})	12	14	40	25
SV (ml)	12	14	40	25
C(a−$\bar{v}$)O$_2$ (ml·100^{-1} ml)	8	2	10	5
BV (L)	2	0	10	3
Cap. Density in Mus.	2	?	55	?
Mus. Oxid. Enzymes	40	?	160	?

$\dot{V}O_2$ max = aerobic capacity
$\dot{Q}_{CO}$ = cardiac output
SV = stroke volume
C(a−$\bar{v}$)O$_2$ = arterial minus mixed venous oxygen content
BV = blood volume
Cap. Density = capillary density in skeletal muscle, ie the number of capillaries per muscle fiber.
Mus. Oxid. = skeletal muscle oxidative enzyme content

(Adapted from Knuttgen, Personal Communication, April 1981)

after two to three years of regular aerobic exercise. The opportunity for checking these possibilities, however, should provide a stimulus for longitudinal investigation. At this juncture, it is postulated that men and women adapt in a similar fashion to regular exercise.

Physiological "improvement" presumably comes about only with exposure to overload. The intensity of exercise readily tolerated is dependent on genetic endowment and initial physical condition. An upward adjustment in exercise intensity is necessary as physical fitness improves. In general, an exercise intensity in excess of 50% of aerobic capacity is usually necessary to demonstrate physiological "improvement" or adaptation. Such a program carried out for one hour, three times per week, constitutes about the minimum amount of exercise (for an otherwise relatively sedentary person) necessary to achieve measurable physiological changes. Walking rapidly would meet the 50% $\dot{V}O_2$ max criterion for most relatively sedentary people.

Summary

This contribution was prepared to provide a "broad brush" background in physiology for those interested in relationships between diet and exercise. It was not intended to serve as a comprehensive review. Initially, attention was focused on conceptual differences among exercise, physical conditioning, and training. It was emphasized that for skeletal muscle adaptation to take place, the muscle must regularly contract against greater than normal loads (overload principle). The various types of muscle contraction were identified and the point was made that muscular adaptation tends to be task specific. Walking is represented as a simple but useful regular exercise that most people can enjoy. Some of the patterns of fuel utilization during exercise are presented, as is an outline summary of some of the most important physiological effects of regular exercise. A final table illustrates some of the effects of exercise carried out for two to three months or two to three years by those who are young adults or middle-aged. Emphasis is placed on cardiovascular and skeletal muscle variables.

Acknowledgments

I wish to thank Patricia MacKeen and Joseph Loomis for their editorial suggestions and Becky Nilson for typing the manuscript.

References

1. Bligh J, Johnson KG: Glossary of terms for thermal physiology. *J Appl Physiol* 35:941–961, 1973.
2. Hettinger T: *Physiology of Strength*. Springfield, IL, Thomas, 1961.
3. Buskirk ER: Temperature regulation with exercise, in Hutton RS (ed): *Exercise and Sports Sciences Reviews*, vol 5. Santa Barbara, CA, Journal Publishing Affiliates, 1977, pp 45–88.
4. Knuttgen HG: Force, work, power, exercise. *Med Sci Sports* 10:227–228, 1978.
5. Committee on Dietary Allowances, Food and Nutrition Board: *Recommended Dietary Allowances*. Washington, DC, Division of Biological Sciences, Assembly of Life Sciences, National Research Council, National Academy of Sciences, 1980.
6. Buskirk ER: Problems related to the caloric cost of living. *Bull NY Acad Med* 36:365–388, 1960.
7. Buskirk ER, Mendez J: Energy: Caloric requirements, in Alfin-Slater RB, Kritchevsky D (eds): *Human Nutrition—A Comprehensive Treatise Vol 3A Macronutrients*, chap 2. New York, Plenum Press, 1980, pp 49–95.
8. Rahkila P, Soimarjavi J, Karvinen E, et al: Lipid metabolism during exercise. II. Respiratory exchange ratio and muscle glycogen content during 4h bicycle ergometry in two groups of healthy men. *Eur J Appl Physiol* 45:147–154, 1980.
9. Buskirk ER: Some nutritional considerations in the conditioning of athletes. *Ann Rev Nutr* 1:319–350, 1981.
10. Mole PA, Oscai LB, Holloszy JO: Adaptation of muscle to exercise. Increases in levels of palmityl-CoA synthetase, carnitine palmityl-transferase and palmityl-CoA dehydrogenase, and in the capacity to oxidize fatty acids. *J Clin Invest* 50:2323–2330, 1971.
11. Askew EW, Dohm GL, Huston RL: Fatty acid and ketone body metabolism in the rat: Response to diet and exercise. *J Nutr* 105:1422–1432, 1975.
12. Bransford DR, Howley ET: Effects of training on plasma FFA during exercise in women. *Eur J Appl Physiol* 41:151–158, 1979.
13. Nikkila EA, Taskinen MR, Ruhunen S, et al: Lipoprotein lipase activity in adipose tissue and skeletal muscle of runners: Relation to serum lipoproteins. *Metabolism* 27:1661–1671, 1978.
14. Ingjer F, Brodal P: Capillary supply of skeletal muscle fibers in untrained and endurance-trained women. *Eur J Appl Physiol* 38:291–299, 1978.
15. Astrand PO, Rodahl K: *Textbook of Work Physiology: Physiological Basis of Exercise*. New York, McGraw-Hill, 1977, pp 394–396.
16. Shepherd JT, Vanhoutte PM: *The Human Cardiovascular System*. New York, Raven Press, 1979, pp 156–179.
17. Grande F, Taylor H: Adaptive changes in the heart, vessels and patterns of control under chronically high loads, in Hamilton WF (ed): *Handbook of Physiology—Circulation III*, chap 74. Washington, DC, Am Physiol Soc, 1965, pp 2615–2677.
18. Rowell LB: Human cardiovascular adjustments to exercise and thermal stress. *Physiol Rev* 54:75–159, 1974.
19. Nadel ER, Stolwijk JAJ: Sweat gland response to the efferent thermoregulatory signal. *Arch Sci Physiol* 27:A67–A77, 1973.
20. Stolwijk JAJ, Nadel ER: Thermoregulation during positive and negative work exercise. *Fed Proc* 32:1607–1613, 1973.

21. Hartley LH: Growth hormone and catecholamine response to exercise in relation to physical training. *Med Sci Sports* 7:34–36, 1975.

22. Hartley LH, Mason JW, Hogan RP, et al: Multiple hormonal responses to graded exercise in relation to physical training. *J Appl Physiol* 33:602–606, 1972.

23. Bloom SR, Johnson RH, Park DM, et al: Differences in the metabolic and hormonal response to exercise between racing cyclists and untrained individuals. *J Physiol* 258:1–18, 1976.

24. Terjung RL, Winder WW: Exercise and thyroid function. *Med Sci Sports* 7:20–26, 1975.

PHYSICAL ACTIVITY AND DIETARY INTAKES

Nathan J. Smith, MD*

Energy Balance

The Ten State National Nutrition Survey, conducted in the United States a little more than ten years ago, was the first attempt to look at the nutrition status of a population in a modern industrial society.[1] Since that time, many industrialized nations have also conducted nutrition surveys. Nutrition problems, now well documented, are similar in all of industrialized societies and have not changed significantly since the original United States survey in 1970. Monitoring of nutrition status of the United States population has continued.

Health problems related to nutrition, that can be considered to be of significance in populations living with economic affluence, mechanization, and food abundance, are primarily problems that result from imbalances in energy intakes and expenditures. It should not be too surprising that intakes of food energy in excess of need exist in a society where 85% to 90% of the population can afford to purchase many times their required amount of food. This is particularly likely when opportunities for spontaneous energy expenditure are severely restricted in the mechanized, urban environments where most individuals live. Obesity is the inevitable result of having energy intakes exceed energy expenditures and is the most prevalent of these nutrition-related health problems. This, of course, depends on whether or not one is willing to accept the concept that obesity as a public health problem has something to do with nutrition and food energy intakes.

The prevalence of obesity is impossible to define since it is not possible to state precisely the degree of fatness that constitutes obesity. It is quite obvious from the current data on the weight of children in the United States that a significant percentage of them are excessively heavy and can be judged to be obese. If one reviews the current data from the National Center for Health Statistics, a skewing of the distribution curve of children's weights to the heavy side becomes readily apparent by the age of four or five.[2] This is apparent by comparing the distance of the fifth and ninety-fifth percentiles from the fiftieth percentile. In a normal Gaussian distribution, the fifth and ninety-fifth percentiles are of equal distance from the fiftieth percentile. As expected, this is true for the distribution of children's heights at all ages. However, as can be seen in Figure 1, the ninety-fifth percentile for weight of adolescents who are 14 years old is nearly twice the distance from the fiftieth percentile as is the fifth percentile. This skewed distribution is present at all ages after the age of three.

---

*University of Washington School of Medicine, Seattle, Washington.

**Distribution of Height and Weight
of 10 Year Old Boys**

Percentile	5	50	95
Weight (Kg.)	24.3	31.4	45.2
Height (cm)	127.7	137.5	148.0

Figure 1. The distribution of height and weight as gathered from subjects in the United States (National Center for Health Statistics). The fifth and ninety-fifth percentiles for height are approximately equal distance from the fiftieth percentile whereas the distribution of weights has the ninety-fifth percentile twice as far from the fiftieth as the fifth percentile, indicating a striking excess of body weight, over fatness in this population. (NCHS Growth Charts, National Center for Health Statistics, 1976)[2]

The problem of energy imbalance is of concern to the pediatrician. Although it is difficult to document the health handicaps of obesity, there is good documentation that obesity has adverse social consequences in our society, especially for the young. Current epidemiologic data on obesity demonstrate that the population at greatest risk in the adult segment of society is the high-income married male with a college degree, military service, and entering a professional career. All of these life events are associated with an increasing risk of obesity.

Energy Intake

In contrast to problems of energy intakes in excess of expenditures, inadequate dietary energy is a common occurrence. It is known that approximately 15% of the population in this country lives at a level of poverty that does not allow them to satisfy normal food energy needs. Children in these circumstances do not have problems of excess intakes of food energy but have energy imbalances resulting from *involuntary* energy deprivation. In current data on the size of children, it is well documented that there is a correlation between small body size and levels of poverty. This is due in large part to the limited availability of food energy during periods of demanding growth. The involuntary energy deprivation of poverty during adolescence, when food energy demands are the greatest, may also have potentially adverse behavioral consequences, particularly in a society dominated by food excess. Such effects are certainly unpleasant to contemplate.

At the opposite end of the spectrum, we find inadequate energy intakes in children and adolescents due to *completely voluntary* restriction of caloric intake. This is a common occurrence in the adolescent girl who finds herself in a sedentary existence and must voluntarily restrict her energy intake to little more than a basal level in order to avoid obesity, a social disaster that can't be tolerated.

The consequences of either involuntary or voluntary intakes of inadequate energy by young people in this country can be documented with varying degrees of sophistication. Failure to satisfy one's genetic growth potential has been mentioned as a problem among the poor. The underfunctioning of the underfed older child who is in negative energy balance is less well documented. It has been well demonstrated that the efficiency of students who omit breakfast is decreased when tested in midmorning both in academic work and in tests of physical performance. Inadequate energy intakes prompt even more sedentary behavior which, for the young girl, demands further restriction of caloric intake. This may serve to further reduce interest and ability to be active and, until recently, contributed to a highly disturbing level of inactivity among large numbers of adolescent girls.

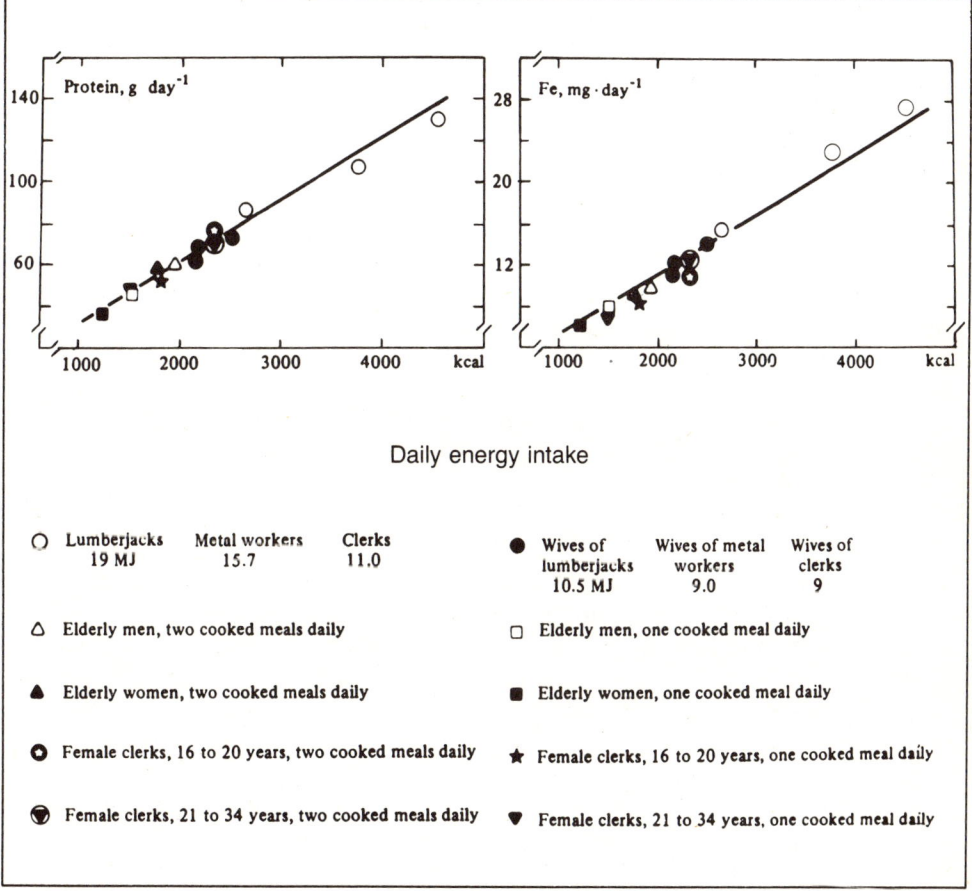

Figure 2. The dietary intake of two essential nutrient substances in relationship to caloric intake which relates to the energy expenditure of the different population groups. Energy expenditure and a moderate energy change is essential for a satisfactory intake of essential nutrients. Reproduced with permission from Astrand P-O: *Int Med* 1:25, 1979.[3] (Courtesy of Franklin Scientific Publications, London)

In addition to the decreased vitality of sedentary young girls, the markedly restricted energy intakes generate a concern for the adequacy of intakes of essential nutrients. Most of the essential nutrients have a rather stable concentration in a mixed American diet that parallels closely the caloric density of that diet. For example, the iron content of an American or western European diet will be approximately six milligrams per thousand calories. This energy-nutrient relationship is evident in data on the energy intakes of individuals with varying levels of energy expenditure. Figure 2 demonstrates the effect of varying levels of caloric intake on the intake of protein and iron. There is an obvious, close straight line relationship between energy intake and the intake of these two essential nutrients.[3] Many women have an energy exchange that allows iron intakes that are inadequate to meet their calculated needs. The caloric intakes of a large number, perhaps the majority, of adolescent girls from middle and upper income families are much less than the food energy intakes of the subjects studied in these experiments. It is not surprising that recent national and regional nutrition surveys of populations of school-aged children in the United States document clearly that adolescent girls are at greatest risk of inadequate intakes of essential nutrients.[4]

It is evident from even a more cursory inquiry that neither energy expenditure nor energy intake of a young person or an adult can be quantitated confidently on a daily basis. Diet records and 24-hour recalls are qualitative instruments at best. The analysis of a large number of 24-hour diet recall records compiled by professional nutritionists from a population of high school girls a few years ago revealed a median caloric intake of 1165 kilocalories (kcal). This energy intake, if truly reflecting the actual energy intake, would be incompatible with life. There was, obviously, significant under-reporting of food intakes.

Energy Expenditure

With limited ability to evaluate caloric intakes, how can we measure expenditures? The most reliable measure of energy expenditure is through quantitation of oxygen consumption. This has been done with humans living in a human calorimeter under very artificial living conditions or involved in certain typical activities while wearing some apparatus such as a Douglas Bag, that can deliver oxygen and collect exhaled carbon dioxide quantitatively. Currently available electronic pulse monitors can provide important semiquantitative data on the energy expenditure of children which are more precise than direct observation or the scoring of movies that have been used to assess energy expending behavior in the past.

Several groups of investigators studied populations of school boys and girls in whom oxygen consumption was measured at rest and then pulse rates were monitored during typical daily activies.[5] Total energy expenditures have been generally judged to be low, actually lower than recommended energy intakes for these age groups. It is interesting that energy expenditures in these studies were no different for the leanest and the fattest children. Thin children, for example, did not expend more energy while sitting in class than did the children who were heavier. More recently, Spady estimated the energy expenditure of 37 children, nine and ten years of age, during daily activities by measuring resting oxygen consumption and pulse rate monitoring. The mean total energy expended during a school day for 22 boys in the study was 2,100 kcal; for the 15 girls, it was 1,700 kcal. The recommended intakes were 2,500 kcal and 2,300 kcal, respectively.

Without attempting to directly measure energy expenditure, several investigators have attempted to define physical activity patterns of children by monitoring heart rates. In a Belgium study of 11 active 12 year-old boys, it was found that during summer holiday, only 3% of their time was spent in an activity that produced a moderate increase in pulse rate; at no time during the several days of monitoring did they take part in heavy, intense or vigorous activity.[7] In another study, 12 year-old children were found to experience heart rates greater than 176 beats per minute for no more than four to six minutes a day.

A series of studies of particular interest are those of Gilliam et al at the University of Michigan.[8] During the summer vacation period, they monitored the pulse rates of 40 children, six and seven years old, living in small communities in Michigan with populations of approximately 5,000 each. The boys and girls had heart rates greater than 160 per minute for only 20 minutes and 9 minutes, respectively, during each 12-hour period of monitoring. Gilliam et al concluded that their data, along with that of others, demonstrate that children who live in environments conducive to moderate physical activity seldom experience heart rates of sufficient intensity to promote desired cardiovascular fitness. Recognizing that physical activity has been reported to reduce the incidence of obesity, increase high density lipoprotein cholesterol (HDL), decrease triglyceride values, decrease systolic blood pressure, and reduce resting heart rate, these investigators question whether patterns of minimal physical exercise and low energy expenditures should not be viewed as a major health concern.

Increased energy expenditure has not been a prominent part of weight control programs in the past. This may, in part, be due to the fact that only recently have studies shown that obese individuals, as a group, have energy intakes that are not measurably different in relation to energy expenditure from that of lean individuals.

Even the most carefully conducted studies fail to demonstrate a relationship between an individual's energy expenditure and energy intake. Edholm measured energy expenditure and energy intakes over a period of 14 days in 12 military cadets who were healthy and whose weights were stable.[9] When plotting the daily energy intake versus the daily energy expenditure, it would be reasonable to expect a straight line relationship. This certainly doesn't happen in any 24-hour period. Even if the total 14-day intake is plotted against expenditure, only two of the twelve cadets' energy intakes and expenditures begin to approximate each other. In spite of these kinds of data, a carefully regulated energy balance must exist for most individuals since most adult individuals maintain a rather remarkably stable weight. The healthy young male cadets in Edholm's study had stable weights but the mechanism responsible for maintaining their energy balance is unknown. This mechanism, whatever it might be, obviously works most effectively in the presence of reasonable energy exchanges of 2,500 to 3,000 kcal for adolescents, and not much less for young adults.

Nutrient Requirements

Controlling energy balance is often difficult; however, it is also difficult to provide an adequate intake of essential nutrients on the low energy intakes that must accompany low energy expenditures. Many essential nutrients, especially minerals, are distributed widely in our food supply, but in low concentration. It is, therefore, difficult and often impossible to assure nutritional adequacy of diets that are low in energy content. Adequate essential nutrients may not be available in diets of less than 2,000 kcal for adults and adolescents.

The problem of obtaining an adequate intake of essential nutrients on low energy diets has been documented in relation to iron intakes in adolescent girls and in older women during their reproductive years. Where there is markedly reduced energy expenditure, high motivation to avoid obesity and, thus, markedly limited caloric intakes, inadequate intakes of iron are likely to occur.

In recent years, quantitative studies of the concentration of iron in the US diet and its bioavailability have allowed precise estimates of dietary sources of iron in relation to the energy content of the diet. In addition, quantitation of iron intakes, losses, and distribution in the body have allowed rather precise identification of iron requirements. With these data at hand, the recommended dietary iron allowance for menstruating women is 18.0 mg per day,[10] an allowance also recommended during adolescent growth. This suggests that the iron intake of almost all healthy adolescents and menstruating women could be satisfied on a quality diet of 3000 kcal with each 1000 calories containing 6.0 mg of dietary iron. As this is a dietary allowance judged to be adequate to meet the needs of practically all healthy individuals, and not a requirement, large numbers of individuals may not require this large intake of iron.

The determining factor for iron requirements in women between 12 and 50 years of age is, obviously, their individual iron losses with menstruation. Several years ago, Halberg et al[11] documented these losses in a population of healthy girls, 15 years of age, by collecting and quantitating menstrual iron losses over a period of several months. Two important facts were derived from this study. First, there was essentially a tenfold variation among the girls in the amount of iron lost in a given menstrual period. Secondly, Halberg's studies documented that there was a high degree of consistency in the amount of iron that was lost month after month by an individual. The girls with larger than average iron losses were consistently losing larger amounts and were, therefore, at greatest risk of becoming iron depleted and iron deficient. The frequency with which iron deficiency develops in menstruating females will depend, to a large degree, on their intake of dietary iron; this will be directly related to the energy content of the diet. If the iron intake is to be generous and excess energy intake avoided, it is obvious that there must be a reasonable energy expenditure.

In order to assess iron deficiency related to menstrual iron losses and the requirements of adolescent growth, erythrocyte protoporphyrin levels were used as an indicator of iron depletion in a population of women in the state of Washington. It was found that 20% of adolescent girls and women are not meeting their needs for dietary iron. Only about 8% of this population had detectable anemia. In the population of girls 12 to 16 years of age, the problem is not income-related. In the adult population, low-income women with earlier and more frequent pregnancies, less medical attention, and lower total dietary intakes, have a greater prevalence of iron deficiency. Low-income adolescent males are also at risk of iron depletion with their high requirements for iron due to adolescent growth and with limited access to sufficient amounts of food in poverty households.[12]

Nutrition and Human Performance

There is increased interest in the problem of iron deficiency with the documentation of the clinical significance of iron depletion without any evidence of detectable anemia. Compromised athletic performance of young women participating in varsity sports programs was noted to be associated with biochemical evidence of iron depletion but without detectable anemia. The experiments of Finch et al[13] are pertinent to this clinical observation. The study involved rats with a stable and identical level of hemoglobin, having been fed either iron-deficient or control diets, with or without supplemental iron. The iron-deficient animals, without anemia, showed striking limitation in exercise capacity which promptly responded to iron therapy. This limited exercise ability was associated with a striking increase in blood lactate levels and a rather precipitous fall in pH. These changes were found to be a consequence of limited aerobic carbohydrate metabolism and an early reliance on anaerobic energy production with resultant lactate accumulation and fatigue. Alpha gylcerophosphate dehydrogenase is the iron-dependent enzyme function most compromised.

Studies of nine women athletes with no anemia, but with low transferrin saturation and plasma ferritin values, showed findings of lactate accumulation similar to the rat studies. The post-exercise lactate levels were normal when the athletes were retested following two weeks of iron therapy which had completely normalized their iron assessment values. These studies, along with the rat experiments, indicate that iron plays a significant role in oxidative energy metabolism unrelated to the presence or absence of anemia.

Our experience in sports medicine in recent years has drawn attention to the problems of energy balance, particularly in the young. The most prevalent nutrition-related problems among young athletes, as in the general population, are problems related to satisfying energy needs. Large numbers of young athletes fail to satisfy the high energy demands of vigorous training. There will be those from poverty backgrounds who have little or no food available to them. There are young athletes from the more affluent, but highly disorganized families, that likewise fail to have an adequate diet available in the home. There is also the highly intent individual, ie, the overcommitted young student with academic, social, and athletic commitments that "doesn't have time to eat" and will most likely have inadequate intakes of energy. These factors contribute to the common problem of the underfed athlete and prompts the truism that when the athlete underperforms, ascertain whether he or she is getting enough to eat.

The problem of excess energy intakes will likewise be encountered in the sports medicine clinic, particularly among participants in low energy expending sports where minimal levels of body fat are highly desired for optimal performance. These include the athletes involved in women's diving, gymnastics, and figure skating. Advising the young gymnast who is spending six or more hours training in the gym daily that additional exercise is needed to decrease body fat is an appropriate message to correct a common problem.

Vigorous exercise, as frequently experienced with athletic training, does not significantly increase the dietary needs for any specific nutrient. As high energy demands are satisfied, there will be a concomitant increase in nutrient intakes. Increased energy expenditures through exercise will also be conducive to maintenance of energy balance.

References

1. *Ten-State Nutrition Survey*, Washington DC. US Department of Health, Education, and Welfare Publication (HSM) 72–8132, 1972.
2. *NCHS Growth Charts*, Monthly vital statistics report 25 (3), suppl (HRA 76–1120), Rockville, MD, National Center for Health Statistics 1976.
3. Astrand PO: Diet and exercise: how to secure an adequate intake of essential nutrients. *Int Med* 1:23–26, 1979.
4. Hodges RE, Krehl WA: Nutritional status of teenagers in Iowa. *Am J Clin Nutr* 17:200–211, 1965.
5. Bradfield RB: Determination of daily energy expenditure in the field. *Am J Clin Nutr* 24:1148–1154, 1971.
6. Spady DW: Total daily energy expenditure of healthy free ranging school children. *Am J Clin Nutr* 33:766–775, 1980.
7. Seliger V, Trefny Z, Barfunkar S, et al: The habitual activity and physical fitness of twelve year old boys. *Acta Pediatr Belg* 28:54–59, 1974.
8. Gilliam TB, Freedson PS, Greenen DL, et al: Physical activity patterns determined by heart rate in 6–7 year old children. *Med Sci Sports Exerc* 13:65–67, 1981.
9. Edholm OG, Adam JM, Healy MJR, et al: Food intake and energy expenditure of army recruits. *Am J Clin Nutr* 24:1091–1107, 1971.
10. *Recommended Dietary Allowances*, ed 9. Washington, DC, Food and Nutrition Board, National Research Council, National Academy of Sciences, 1980.
11. Halberg L, Hogdahl AM, Nilsson L, et al: Menstrual blood loss. *Acta Obstet Gynec Scandinav* 45:320–351, 1966.
12. Cook JD, Finch CA, Smith NJ: Assessing iron status of a population. *Am J Clin Nutr* 32:2115–2123, 1979.
13. Finch CA, Miller LR, Inamdar AR, et al: Iron deficiency in the rat. Physiologic and biochemical studies of muscle dysfunction. *J Clin Invest* 58:447–453, 1976.

INTERRELATION OF PHYSICAL ACTIVITY AND NUTRITION

Moderators: Stanley M. Garn, PhD
Fellow, Center For Human Growth and Development
Professor of Nutrition
University of Michigan
Ann Arbor, Michigan

and

Richard J. Jones, MD
Director, Division of Scientific Policy
Secretary, Council on Scientific Affairs
American Medical Association
Chicago, Illinois

INTERRELATION OF PHYSICAL ACTIVITY AND NUTRITION ON LIPID METABOLISM*

Peter D. Wood, DSc, PhD**
William L. Haskell, PhD**

The purpose of this paper is to examine some major aspects of the influence of increased physical activity level and concomitant dietary intake upon human lipid metabolism. Attention will be focused on plasma lipoprotein concentrations since these are commonly measured and have been strongly associated with risk of future coronary heart disease (CHD) and stroke. The discussion relates largely to populations in developed countries where overnutrition (rather than undernutrition) is a major problem, and where the more vigorous types of physical activity carried out are likely to be recreational (jogging, cycling, swimming, tennis playing), rather than occupational.

Characteristics of Active People

Until recently, individuals who are chronically active in developed countries were in the minority; but in the last five years, increasing numbers of people have adopted a more vigorously active lifestyle, usually by increased participation in leisure time sports.[1] There is evidence from prospective studies[2,3] that such sports participation in some way confers reduced risk of CHD.

Examination of groups of men and women who have taken up vigorous sports reveals a number of characteristic features, of which three are relevant to the present topic: leanness, an increased caloric consumption, and an advantageous plasma lipoprotein distribution.

Leanness. Numerous studies[4] have indicated the tendency for very active groups to show lower relative weights (in relation to "ideal" weight for height and sex) and lower percentages of total body weight as fat, compared to relatively sedentary controls. The marked leanness of middle-aged male and female long-distance runners is shown by way of illustration in Figure 1.

Caloric Consumption. Study of the interrelations of activity level, leanness and caloric intake leads to some conclusions that are readily acceptable to most people. However, other conclusions may also be drawn that appear to be paradoxical. That very active people are lean is visually obvious and seldom disputed. That very active people consume more calories than sedentary people is sometimes doubted ("exercise blunts the appetite"), but is fairly readily accepted. That lean people frequently eat more than obese people follows from

---
*The paper was presented by Dr. Wood.
**Stanford University School of Medicine, Stanford, California

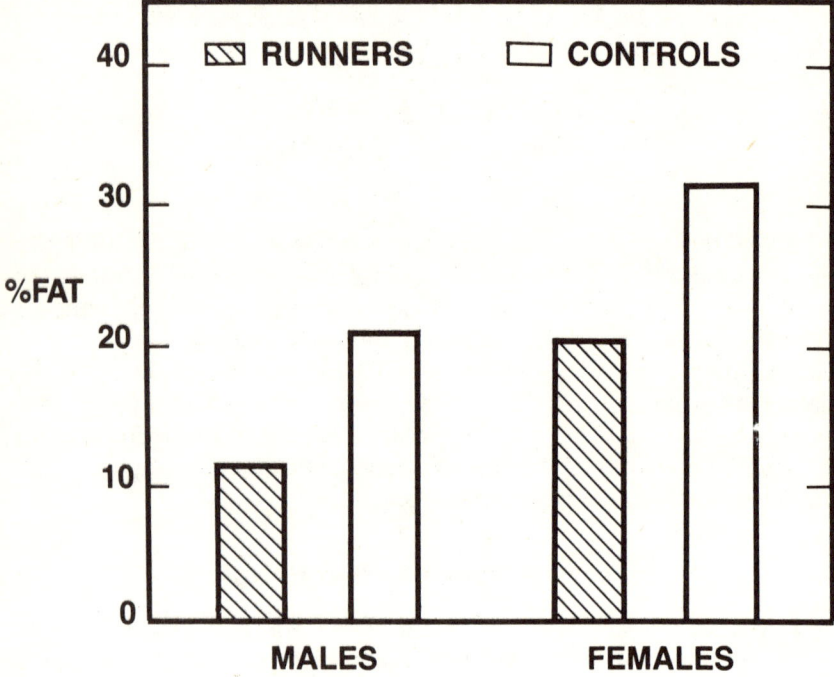

Figure 1. Body fat content (as per cent of total body weight) by hydrostatic weighing for middle-aged male (n = 41) and female (n = 43) long-distance runners, and for control groups of relatively sedentary men and women of similar age, as recorded in the literature. (Reproduced with permission from Wood PD et al: Plasma lipoprotein distributions in male and female runners. *Ann NY Acad Sci* 301:755,1977).

the previous statements, but is far less readily accepted by the public. The lack of consensus on the latter conclusion is probably due to the stereotype of the obese individual being gluttonous.

Many studies have documented, through dietary recall or dietary records, that active individuals eat more than sedentary individuals, all other factors being equal. For instance, our study of middle-aged runners[5] showed an increased daily caloric intake of about 600 kilocalories (kcal) per day for both males and females versus sedentary controls which, allowing 100 kcal per mile run, adequately covered the average reported mileage of six miles per day. Table 1 shows self-reported data for mean dietary intake of dedicated male and female tennis players compared with sedentary controls.[6] Again, total caloric intake is significantly higher for the active group. The calorie intake difference for active and inactive women is particularly striking, and reflects the extreme sedentary life-style of the controls versus the vigorous tennis play (11.2 hrs/week) by the active group.

Table 1. Self-Reported Daily Dietary Intake of Tennis Players and Sedentary Subjects

	Males		Females	
	Tennis (n = 21)	Sedentary (n = 73)	Tennis (n = 22)	Sedentary (n = 49)
Absolute Quantities				
Calories	2726 ± 541*	2450 ± 755	2417 ± 560†	1490 ± 483
Total fat (g)	125 ± 31*	112 ± 47	117 ± 40†	68 ± 29
Saturated fat (g)	48 ± 13*	43 ± 20	44 ± 16†	25 ± 13
Polyunsaturated fat (g)	22 ± 6*	18 ± 10	21 ± 9†	12 ± 7
P/S fat ratio	0.48	0.47	0.50	0.59
Cholesterol (mg)	439 ± 123	474 ± 291	434 ± 222†	315 ± 260
Alcohol (g)	17 ± 19	16 ± 21	19 ± 19	9 ± 16
Nutrients/1000 kcal				
Protein (g)	37 ± 4	41 ± 11	36 ± 5*	43 ± 15
Carbohydrate (g)	98 ± 16	96 ± 27	94 ± 20	96 ± 27
Total fat (g)	46 ± 5	45 ± 10	48 ± 8	45 ± 11
Saturated fat (g)	18 ± 2	17 ± 5	18 ± 4	16 ± 6
Polyunsaturated fat (g)	9 ± 2*	7 ± 3	9 ± 2	8 ± 4
Cholesterol (mg)	161 ± 30	204 ± 140	175 ± 65	209 ± 157
Alcohol (g)	7 ± 8	6 ± 8	8 ± 7*	6 ± 10

Values are mean ± SD
* $p < 0.05$
† $p < 0.001$
(Reproduced with permission from *Metabolism*.[6])

Studies of entire populations have indicated that there is a tendency for obese people to eat less than lean people, although this may not be true in cases of gross obesity. For instance, in a study of three populations in the London area, Keen et al[7] found highly significant inverse correlations between food energy intake and adiposity for both sexes in all three populations. The relationship extended across the whole range of nutrient intake and body mass index.

Several prospective population studies have demonstrated that reported increased caloric consumption is negatively associated with future CHD, eg, those of Morris et al,[8] Yano et al,[9] and of Gordon et al.[10] It has been suggested that the common cause of both increased caloric consumption and decreased CHD is increased exercise level.

Plasma Lipoprotein Pattern. A characteristic pattern of lipoproteins has been observed for active groups versus inactive groups.[11] The major features of the plasma pattern (relative to sedentary controls) are decreased concentrations of triglycerides, low-density lipoprotein (LDL) cholesterol and, often, total cholesterol; and increased concentrations of high-density lipoprotein (HDL) cholesterol. Examples of group differences are given in Table 2 for middle-aged male and female runners and for younger elite runners, versus random controls.

Since LDL-cholesterol concentrations are directly and HDL-cholesterol concentrations are inversely related to risk of developing CHD,[12] more active groups generally show a plasma lipoprotein pattern that is clearly advantageous with respect to CHD risk. The association of increased physical activity with this lipoprotein pattern has generally been found to be independent of most other factors, although there is a distinct possibility that the concomitant leanness may also be an influencing factor.

Nature of the Active Person's Diet

Since it is clear that active individuals generally consume more total calories per unit of body mass than sedentary individuals, the interesting question arises: "What do they choose to eat more of?" When this question relates to free-living groups, rather than to athletes at a training table, the answer appears to be "more of the same," at least in US populations. Our studies of middle-aged runners have indicated that the qualitative nature of their increased caloric intake was generally the same as that of randomly selected controls: cholesterol intake per 1000 kcal, saturated or polyunsaturated fat per 1000 kcal, and alcohol intake per 1000 kcal were all essentially the same in runners and controls. Table 1 demonstrates the same findings for tennis players versus sedentary controls.[6] Total calories, saturated fat and polyunsaturated fat consumption were all higher in the tennis players, but generally the *proportions* of nutrients within the overall diet were not significantly different. A recent study by Hartung et al[13] found that middle-aged male marathon runners and joggers were not different from inactive men in qualitative dietary habits. It therefore appears that active people eat and drink more than sedentary people, and that they choose a similar variety of foods so that the qualitative nature of the diets for the two groups is much the same.

Table 2. Plasma Lipid and Lipoprotein Cholesterol Concentrations* and Ratios in Runners and Controls

	Runners (Age 35–59)		Random Controls (Age 30–59)		Elite male runners (age 21–34) (n = 20)	Random male controls (age 26–30) (n = 72)
	Males (n = 41)	Females (n = 43)	Males (n = 743 or 145†)	Females (n = 934 or 101#)		
Triglycerides (mg/100 ml)	70 ± 24§	56 ± 19§	146 ± 105	123 ± 89	74 ± 25§	92 ± 37
Total cholesterol (mg/100 ml)	200 ± 22§	193 ± 33§	212 ± 38	209 ± 38	175 ± 26§	189 ± 36
Cholesterol in (mg/100 ml):						
LDL	125 ± 21§	113 ± 33§	139 ± 32	124 ± 34	108 ± 25§	124 ± 36
HDL	64 ± 13§	75 ± 14§	43 ± 10	56 ± 14	56 ± 12§	49 ± 11
VLDL	11	7	28	28	11	15
Ratio: HDL/LDL cholesterol	0.51	0.66	0.31	0.45	0.56	0.39
Ratio: Total cholesterol/HDL cholesterol	3.1	2.6	4.9	3.7	3.1	3.9

* mean ± SD
† n = 145 for LDL-, HDL- and VLDL-cholesterol concentrations
# n = 101 for LDL-, HDL-, and VLDL-cholesterol concentrations
§ Mean for runners is significantly different ($p \leq 0.05$) from appropriate control group.
(Reproduced with permission from *Lipids*.[11])

The Influence of Diet on Plasma Lipoproteins

The effect of dietary composition on plasma lipoprotein concentrations is well established in some areas, but less so in others. Diets relatively high in saturated fat and cholesterol generally tend to result in relatively high plasma concentrations of LDL-cholesterol, and hence of total cholesterol. Diets high in polyunsaturated fat, and diets characterized as "high carbohydrate—low-fat—low-cholesterol" tend to result in low LDL-cholesterol and low total cholesterol concentrations. Thus, transfer from a "typical" American diet to a vegetarian diet (especially one without eggs), usually results in a fall in plasma total cholesterol and in LDL-cholesterol concentration.

Dietary influences on the important risk predictor, HDL-cholesterol concentration, are less clear except for the increased plasma HDL-cholesterol levels associated with alcohol consumption.[14] High fat diets seem to elevate HDL-cholesterol as well as LDL-cholesterol, while low-fat diets (Pritikin diet, Tarahumara Indians' diet) are associated with relatively low levels of both LDL-cholesterol and HDL-cholesterol. This effect is illustrated by the study of Knuiman et al,[15] in which plasma total cholesterol and HDL-cholesterol levels were determined in schoolboy populations from 16 countries around the world, from highly developed to relatively undeveloped regions. A wide range of concentrations was found, with a significant correlation coefficient of 0.90 for the relationship between total cholesterol and HDL-cholesterol. The authors concluded that when the total cholesterol is high as a result of the diet consumed, the HDL-cholesterol concentration also tends to be high. The effect of diet is probably clearer between populations than within populations because other determinants of HDL-cholesterol (alcohol intake, physical activity level) may further obscure the effect of diet within populations.

Effects of Exercise on Body Composition, Food Intake and Plasma Lipoprotein Pattern

A recently completed one-year, randomized, controlled training study by our group involved 48 middle-aged sedentary men assigned to exercise (running) and 33 men assigned to remain as sedentary controls.[16] Results indicated that increases in plasma HDL-cholesterol, and decreases in LDL-cholesterol, occurred (relative to controls) only in those men who ran ten miles per week or more on average, for at least nine months. One-year change in HDL-cholesterol in runners was positively correlated with average miles run (Spearman's rho = 0.48, p = 0.006). However, body composition changes occurred in relation to miles run, and one-year change in per cent of body fat was also correlated (negatively) with miles run (rho = −0.47, p = 0.007). Adjustment procedures suggested that running mileage and reduction in body fat were both independently associated with increase in plasma HDL-cholesterol.

Measurements of caloric consumption were also made during this trial. Reported caloric consumption increased with increasing running mileage (rho =

0.48, p = 0.006), and, interestingly, there was a relatively strong *negative* relationship between one-year change in caloric intake and one-year change in per cent body fat (rho = −0.56, p = 0.0008), ie, there was a tendency for the men who lost the most body fat to report the largest increase in caloric consumption. Of course, they were also the men who increased their exercise level the most. These findings provide a longitudinal confirmation of the conclusions (discussed earlier) from cross-sectional studies, that leaner people tend to eat more, exercise more and have higher HDL-cholesterol levels than obese people.

A further intriguing finding was a significant positive correlation for runners between one-year change in caloric intake and one-year change in plasma HDL-cholesterol concentration (rho = 0.35, p = 0.047). Since the quality of the diet consumed by the men as they became more active did not change significantly (consistent with the cross-sectional findings[5]), the conclusion is that an increasing (absolute) consumption of fat is associated with an increasing plasma concentration of the "negative" CHD-risk predictor, HDL-cholesterol, in these men.

An increase in the HDL_2 subfraction of total plasma HDL was found to be responsible for the overall increase in HDL-cholesterol with exercise in this trial. This is also consistent with our cross-sectional finding that dedicated long-distance runners have higher HDL_2 levels in plasma than do sedentary controls.[17] This may relate to the *lower* levels of post-heparin hepatic lipase activity seen in runners versus controls.[18,19]

Summary

This discussion of some recent findings emphasizes that indeed nutrition, physical activity and lipid metabolism are closely related. At times, the degree of intertwining can be quite frustrating for investigators. Carefully designed, long-term studies are required to further separate the effects of changes in body fat and in the level of exercise on plasma lipoprotein concentrations. Meanwhile, there seems little doubt that the vigorously active lifestyle is associated in developed countries with relative leanness, increased caloric consumption, probably increased dietary fat consumption, and a reputedly beneficial plasma lipoprotein pattern. It might be said that very active people maintain a "desirable" plasma lipoprotein pattern in spite of eating, on average, the "typical American diet," and, indeed, in spite of eating *more* of it than do sedentary people. However, we should clearly consider the probability that the lipoprotein pattern of active people (and, in particular, the level of LDL-cholesterol) would be further improved by concomitant improvement in their diet.

Looking to future research, two areas seem to hold particular promise. First, further study is needed of the possibility that the high dietary fat intake that appears to be characteristic of very active people in developed countries may be directly responsible for their elevated plasma HDL-cholesterol levels, rather than the exercise *per se*. Second, the specific influences of dietary fat intake and of increased exercise upon the HDL subfractions (HDL_2 and HDL_3), and of the hepatic lipase—lipoprotein lipase system that seems to control their concentrations, merit further study.

Acknowledgments

Work by the authors and their colleagues, described in this paper, has been supported by NIH grant #HL 24462, and by a gift from Best Foods, a Unit of CPC North America.

References

1. *The Perrier Study: Fitness in America*. New York, Great Waters of France, Inc, 1979.
2. Morris JN, Everitt MG, Pollard R, et al: Vigorous exercise in leisure-time: Protection against coronary heart disease. *Lancet* 2:1207–1210, 1980.
3. Paffenbarger RS, Jr, Wing AL, Hyde RT: Physical activity as an index of heart attack risk in college alumni. *Am J Epidemiol* 108:161–175, 1978.
4. Brownell KD, Stunkard AJ: Physical activity in the development and control of obesity, in Stunkard AJ (ed): *Obesity*. Philadelphia, WB Saunders Company, 1980, pp 300–324.
5. Blair SN, Ellsworth NM, Haskell WL, et al: Comparison of nutrient intake in middle-aged men and women runners and controls. *Med Sci Sports Exerc* 13:310–315, 1981.
6. Vodak PA, Wood PD, Haskell WL, et al: HDL-cholesterol and other plasma lipid and lipoprotein concentrations in middle-aged male and female tennis players. *Metabolism* 29:745–752, 1980.
7. Keen H, Thomas BH, Jarrett RJ, et al: Nutrient intake, adiposity, and diabetes. *Brit Med J* 1:655–658, 1979.
8. Morris JN, Marr JW, Clayton DG: Diet and heart: A postscript. *Brit Med J* 2:1307–1314, 1977.
9. Yano K, Rhoads GG, Kagan A, et al: Dietary intake and the risk of coronary heart disease in Japanese men living in Hawaii. *Am J Clin Nutr* 31:1270–1279, 1978.
10. Gordon T, Kagan A, Garcia-Palmieri M, et al: Diet and its relation to coronary heart disease and death in three populations. *Circulation* 63:500–515, 1981.
11. Wood PD, Haskell WL: The effect of exercise on plasma high density lipoprotein. *Lipids* 14:417–427, 1979.
12. Miller GJ: High density lipoproteins and atherosclerosis. *Ann Rev Med* 31:97–108, 1980.
13. Hartung GH, Farge EJ, Mitchell RE: Effects of marathon running, jogging and diet on coronary risk factors in middle-aged men. *Prev Med* 10:316–323, 1981.
14. Castelli WP, Gordon T, Hjortland MC, et al: Alcohol and blood lipids. *Lancet* 2:153–155, 1977.
15. Knuiman JT, Hermus RJJ, Hautvast JGAJ: Serum total and high density lipoprotein (HDL) cholesterol concentrations in rural and urban boys from 16 countries. *Atherosclerosis* 36:529–537, 1980.
16. Wood PD, Haskell WL, Williams PT, et al: Exercise and plasma lipoproteins: A one-year randomized, controlled trial. Abstract. *Council on Epidemiology Newsletter* 30:20, 1981.
17. Krauss RM, Lindgren FT, Wood PD, et al: Differential increases in plasma high density lipoprotein subfractions and apolipoproteins in runners. Abstract. *Circulation* 56:III-4, 1977.
18. Krauss RM, Wood PD, Giotas C, et al: Heparin-released plasma lipase activities and lipoprotein levels in distance runners. Abstract. *Circulation* 60:II-73, 1979.
19. Tikkanen MJ, Nikkila EA, Kuusi T, et al: Reduction of plasma high-density lipoprotein$_2$ cholesterol and increase of postheparin plasma hepatic lipase activity during progestin treatment. *Clinica Chimica Acta* 115:63–71, 1981.

PROTEIN METABOLISM AND EXERCISE*

Robert Alan Hoerr, MD**
Vernon Robert Young, PhD**
William Joseph Evans, PhD***

Introduction

Increasing numbers of Americans share the view that exercise is beneficial for their general health and participate regularly in various forms of exercise. National and international allowances for dietary protein and amino acids do not make specific recommendations for persons who exercise regularly.[1,2] Because regular exercise is becoming more prevalent in our culture, we will review the relationships between physical activity, protein and amino acid metabolism, and nutrition in human subjects. We will specifically consider the effect of exercise on muscle and body growth and development, the use of protein as a fuel during exercise, and the changes in amino acid metabolism which occur during exercise in muscle and the whole body. Our purpose is to determine if exercising individuals require higher intakes of protein in their diets than are currently recommended for the general population.

Effects of Exercise on Muscle and Body Growth and Development

Studies with human and animal models show that continuous periods of exercise induce muscular hypertrophy, which is accompanied by an overall anabolic effect on body protein metabolism and by an improvement in somatic growth. These changes are brought about in large part by the effect of exercise on skeletal muscle tissue, which comprises 40% of body weight and accounts for 25% to 30% of total body protein turnover in young adults.[3,4] Exercise changes hormone levels in directions which promote muscle anabolism.[5] Exercise patterns change the morphological and enzymatic characteristics of the different muscle fiber types and the types of protein.[6-9] Animal studies demonstrate that regular exercise enhances amino acid transport into muscle cells and increases the rate of incorporation into muscle proteins, including both the sarcoplasmic and fibrillar protein fractions.[10-12] Higher work loads cause changes in the metabolism and content of the nucleic acids (RNA and DNA), and these changes favor increased rates of protein synthesis and growth.

---

*The paper was presented by Dr. Young.
**Massachusetts Institute of Technology, Cambridge, Massachusetts.
***Boston University, Boston, Massachusetts.

The beneficial effects of moderate exercise on general human health have been discussed in detail at this symposium. We wish to call attention to one particular therapeutically-useful effect of moderate exercise in young children recovering from protein-energy malnutrition. In studies carried out at Institute of Nutrition of Central America and Panama (INCAP) by Torun and Viteri (manuscript in preparation), children, aged 2 to 4 years, under treatment for protein-energy malnutrition, were stimulated to be more physically active through a daily program of games that required mild to moderate levels of energy expenditure. Balance and anthropometric data indicate that the more active children grew better in height and in lean body mass than similar children treated in the traditional manner at INCAP (Fig 1). From these results, we conclude that

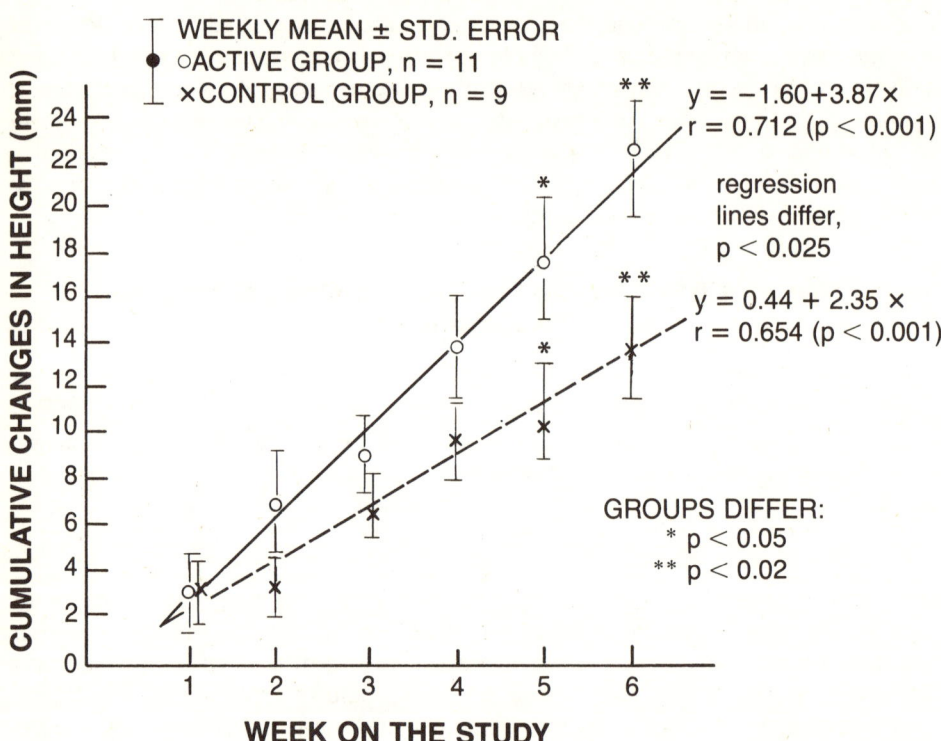

Figure 1. Linear growth in a group of physically active children, as compared with a control group, during recovery from protein-energy malnutrition (PEM). Unpublished data of B. Torun and F. Viteri (INCAP). Reproduced with permission from Young VR, Torun B: *Nutrition in Health and Disease and International Development* (Symposia from the XII International Congress of Nutrition), Harper AE, Davis GK (eds), 1981, p. 79 (Courtesy of Alan R. Liss, Inc)*

*Figures 2 and 3 have been reproduced with permission as above; page nos. are pp. 72 and 73, respectively.

moderate exercise had a growth-enhancing effect and a favorable impact on the utilization of dietary protein. Furthermore, it seems reasonable to expect that this would apply to well-nourished individuals, both children and adults.

Fuels for Muscular Exercise

We will next examine the relative contribution made by protein to the fuel mix which is oxidized for energy production during exercise. The major substrates which comprise this mix include carbohydrates, in the form of muscle glycogen and blood glucose; fat, in the form of free fatty acids; and amino acids, derived from intracellular protein breakdown or from free amino acids. The mix of fuels which is burned during submaximal exercise depends on three main factors: the intensity of the exercise, the degree of conditioning, and the nutritional status of the exercising individual.[13-15] In order to understand how these factors specifically relate to the use of protein as an energy source, we will first describe how they relate to the use of the other fuels, carbohydrate and fat.

Carbohydrate and Fat

The complex interaction between the proteins, actin and myosin, which produces muscle contraction requires energy.[16] This energy comes from the hydrolysis of the high-energy phosphate bonds from either adenosine triphosphate (ATP) or creatine phosphate. Because the concentration of these substances in muscle is small (Table 1), the high energy phosphate bonds must be continuously regenerated if exercise is to continue for a significant period of

Table 1. Stores of Energy in the Normal Adult*

Fuel	Amount	
	kcal	kJ
ATP	1.5	6
Creatine phosphate	3.5	15
Glycogen	1,200	
Fat	140,000	

*From Åstrand[17] and Felig and Wahren.[18] Stores for 20 kg muscle, except for fat (based on total body wt of 75 kg). Reproduced with permission from Young VR, Torun B: *Nutrition in Health and Disease and International Development* (Symposia from the XII International Congress of Nutrition), Harper AE, Davis GK (eds), 1981, p. 57 (Courtesy of Alan R. Liss, Inc)**

**Tables 3–5 have been reproduced with permission as above; page nos. are pp. 70, 71, 67, respectively.

time. Skeletal muscle has a great capacity to regenerate ATP from the anaerobic and oxidative metabolism of both carbohydrate and fat, and together, these fuels provide about 90% of the energy required for exercise.[18-20]

Two of the factors which determine the mix of carbohydrate and fat used during exercise, as mentioned above, are the current state of an individual's training and the intensity of the exercise. Essentially, no matter what the intensity of the exercise, the better trained individual will use fewer carbohydrates, as aerobic training helps skeletal muscle to use free fatty acids. However, as the intensity of the exercise increases, the relative contribution of carbohydrate to the total energy provided increases. When the intensity exceeds the body's maximal ability to take up oxygen ($\dot{V}O_2$ max), skeletal muscle depends almost totally on muscle glycogen stores for its ATP production.[13] The third factor which is important in determining the mix is the diet of the exercising individual. On a high carbohydrate diet, the utilization of carbohydrate increases, and the stores of carbohydrates, as muscle and liver glycogen, increase.[21] On a low carbohydrate diet, the utilization of free fatty acids increases, and carbohydrate stores are reduced.[22]

Protein

The contribution of protein to the fuel mix used during exercise is clearly minor compared to the contribution made by carbohydrate and fat. However, because even small increases in the amount of protein burned may substantially increase the amount of protein required in the diet of an exercising individual, we will consider the studies which have examined this contribution in some detail. Two major experimental approaches have been employed. Earlier studies measured blood and urine levels of nitrogen-containing waste products, especially urea, as indices of the amount of protein which was irreversibly oxidized during exercise. More recent studies have looked at changes in the metabolism of individual amino acids as indices of protein oxidation.

Nitrogen Excretion Studies. The great German chemist Justus Liebig steadfastly maintained that protein was the primary fuel for working muscle.[23] His theory was tested in a number of experiments performed during the last half of the nineteenth century. The most famous of these was conducted by two Zurich professors, Fick and Wisclicenus, who hiked up the Faulhorn in the Bernese Oberland in 1865, collecting their urine for nitrogen analysis before and during their experiment.[24] Unfortunately, they confounded their results by placing themselves on a protein-free diet the day before their climb, thereby certainly reducing their urinary nitrogen excretion. Additionally, by prematurely ending their urine collection on the completion of their descent, any possible post-exercise rise in urinary nitrogen which may have occurred was not detected. They also underestimated their work load. Despite these defects in study design, their urinary nitrogen excretion values demonstrate that protein oxidation would have provided only a small portion of the energy required to make their climb.

The finding that protein is not a major fuel for muscular work was confirmed in a number of other studies, as reviewed in detail by Cathcart[25] and summarized in Table 2. The enhanced urinary nitrogen excretion in these studies was small, indicating that protein oxidation was not the main source of energy. Even so, a rise in urinary nitrogen output frequently occurred on the day of strenuous exercise and for 1 to 2 days thereafter.

The exercise-induced catabolic rise in urinary nitrogen excretion suggests a paradox, since regular exercise promotes an increase in lean body mass and would, therefore, be expected to decrease urinary nitrogen excretion. Several investigators have reexamined urea production and excretion during exercise. Décombaz[26] measured urinary urea clearance by collecting the urine voided by

Table 2. Nineteenth Century Studies on the Effect of Work on Protein Metabolism*

Beigl (1855)	Increased N output following work on a meager diet, but even larger with protein-rich diet.
Smith (1862)	Definite rise in N output on day of 29-mile treadmill walk and day following.
Voit & Pettenkofer (1866)	No effect of work on N output.
Fick and Wisclicenus (1866)	Decreased N output in work urine, post-work urine (but protein-free diet consumed and pre-work control urine reflects normal dietary protein level).
Parkes (1866–1871)	Slightly increased N output both on protein-free diet and mixed diet.
Weigelin (1868)	Increased N output after 2 hrs hard work; rise most pronounced in post-work period.
Schenk (1874)	Data shows slight but definite rise in urea output during work, initial post-work days, though he denied an effect.
Pavy (1876)	Professional pedestrians on ample diet—increased N output on work days compared to rest days.
Flint (1877)	Increased N output with 63.5 miles/day for 5 days.
Breitzcke (1877)	Increased N output in convicts on work days.
Argutinsky (1890)	Increased N output with work, present even when additional energy added bringing diet to adequate total energy supply.
Paton (1891)	Small but definite rise on first and second post-days in a student consuming 3979 kcal, 16 g N.
Krummacher (1896)	Increased N output on post-work days when energy levels 38 and 64 kcal/kg, less when energy increased to 72 kcal/kg.

*Cathcart, EP[25]

11 trained runners after completing a 100 km race. He recorded a net decrease in urea clearance rates during the race and an increase during the following 24 hours. Plasma urea levels were 50% higher after the run and remained elevated for 24 hours. The decline in urea clearance rates accounted for only part of this rise in plasma urea. Urea production rates, inferred from changes in plasma and urinary urea, averaged 44% higher for the race period than pre-race rates. In a similar study, Refsum and Strömme[27] noted a doubling of urea production rates in subjects participating in a 70 km ski race. Haralambie and Berg[28] found that plasma urea levels rose after 60 to 70 minutes in eight groups of subjects studied during various forms of exercise which lasted from 15 minutes to more than 12 hours. The rise correlated with the duration of the exercise. As in the previous two studies, neither a decline in the urea clearance, which decreased 47.6% during a 2 hour bicycle ergometer ride and 56% during a 70 km ski race, could account for the measured rise in plasma urea. Cerny[29] demonstrated that sweat may provide a significant additional route of nitrogen loss during moderate, sustained exercise, which amounted to 0.5 g nitrogen during 2 hours of exercise at 60% to 65% $\dot{V}o_2$ max on a bicycle ergometer. This figure corresponds very closely to the predicted loss of sweat nitrogen that may be extrapolated from the data of Calloway et al[30] for this energy expenditure (8–12 kcal/min). Urea production rates were almost certainly underestimated in the first three studies, since sweat losses were not measured.

These studies demonstrate that sustained moderate to heavy exercise induces an increase in urea production, as well as a decline in urea clearance that is nearly balanced by an increase in sweat urea elimination. Lemon and Mullen[31] estimate, based on their careful review of these and other studies, that proteins may contribute up to 12% of the energy cost of exercise. Poortmans,[32] on the other hand, has calculated that protein catabolism accounts for only about 1% of the energy cost expected during exercise. It is difficult to compare these various experiments since the subjects differed in age, training status, prior dietary history, and duration of exercise, and they were studied in either the fed or post-absorptive state. All of these factors would be expected to alter the metabolic response to exercise. Another factor which may be important in determining the urea response to exercise is the glycogen content of the muscle which, as mentioned earlier, may be manipulated by diet. A higher glycogen content decreases the rise in plasma urea observed during exercise (Fig 2). Some investigators[33] who have employed shorter exercise periods or lower exercise intensities have failed to measure a rise in plasma urea. This may be due to the maintenance of higher muscle glycogen levels in their subjects during the exercise period.

Amino Acid Oxidation Studies. A second approach which has been used to determine the amount of protein used as fuel during exercise has been to measure the oxidation of individual amino acids. Leucine, one of the branched-chain amino acids, has been used as a tracer in these studies because it is an

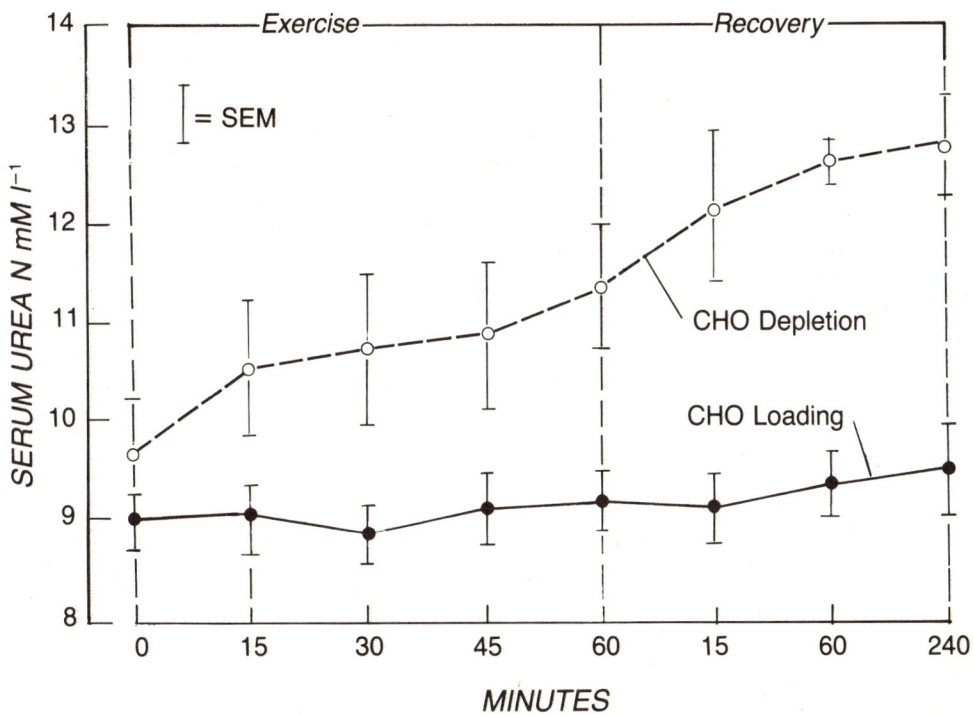

From: LEMON and MULLIN (1980)

Figure 2. Change in serum urea concentration during and following recovery from exercise (for 60 min at 61% $\dot{V}O_2$ max on a bicycle ergometer) in adult male subjects who had received previously a high carbohydrate diet (CHO-loaded) for 3 days or who were carbohydrate depleted. Drawn from Lemon and Mullin.[31] Reproduced with permission. See footnote on page 50.

essential amino acid, and like the other branched-chain amino acids, isoleucine and valine, is present in high concentrations in muscle tissue. Dohm et al[34] have reported that endurance training in rats resulted in an increased oxidation of leucine in muscle tissue, which was accompanied by an increased output of urea nitrogen. Based on these data, he calculated that more than 30% of the energy for muscle contraction can come from proteins.

Since there have been relatively few studies in human subjects designed to quantify changes in whole body amino acid metabolism which occur during exercise, we have begun to explore this problem with the aid of stable isotope probes.[35] Aspects of whole body amino acid metabolism are being measured in adult subjects before and after a 2 hour bicycle ergometer ride at a submaximal intensity. Our preliminary findings reveal that free amino acid levels in venous plasma showed little change in response to exercise, although free fatty acid and glycerol levels, reflective of increased adipose tissue lipolysis, rose during this time. Of course, measurements of plasma amino acid levels may fail to indicate changes in amino acid metabolism that occur during exercise because the plasma level represents the balance between their rates of flow into and out of the circulation. Therefore, using 1-^{13}C-leucine as a stable isotope probe and applying the model described by Waterlow et al,[36,37] we examined whole body leucine kinetics before and during the 2 hour period of moderate exercise. Our initial findings, summarized in Table 3, indicate that a rise in the rate of leucine oxidation, as determined in both trained and untrained subjects who had received only a small breakfast before exercise, was associated with a reduced rate of leucine incorporation into body proteins and a reduced rate of leucine release from body protein breakdown. Using a similar approach, Rennie et al[38] have also observed an increased rate of whole body leucine oxidation although they did not find a reduction in leucine release from body protein breakdown. These investigators have concluded in a more recent paper that the rate of muscle protein breakdown is reduced during exercise.[39]

Table 3. Parameters of Whole Body Leucine Kinetics in Subjects At Rest and During 2 h Exercise at 55% $\dot{V}O_2$ max*

Parameters	Condition		P
	Rest	Exercise	
Leucine Flux	120.4 ± 6.2(15)†	97.0 ± 7.13(15)	< 0.001
Leucine Oxidation	14.8 ± 1.3(8)	46.1 ± 9.7(8)	< 0.01
Leucine Incorporation into protein	113.2 ± 5.4(8)	58.2 ± 9.5(8)	< 0.01

*Unpublished data of Wright, Evans, Phinney and Young (1981).
†Values are μmole.kg^{-1}h^{-1}. Mean ± SEM. Number of subjects in parentheses.
Reproduced with permission. See footnote on p. 51.

Table 4. Contribution of Protein Oxidation† to Total Energy Expenditure‡ (%) at Rest and During 2 Hours of Exercise at 55% $\dot{V}O_2$ max*

Subjects	No.	Pre-Exercise	During Exercise
Untrained	3	14.1	4.8
Trained	5	12.2	2.9

*Unpublished data of Wright et al. (1981)
†Based upon leucine content in whole body protein of 590 μmol g and mean values for leucine oxidation of 14.8 μmol.kg^{-1}h^{-1} (pre-exercise) and 46.1 μmol.kg^{-1}h^{-1} (during exercise).
‡Total energy expenditure derived from indirect calorimetry using measured values of VO_2 and "R" during a 2 h period.
Reproduced with permission. See footnote on p. 51.

How does the increased oxidation of leucine relate to the substantial increase in total energy expenditure during exercise? We have calculated that the contribution made by amino acid catabolism to the total energy expenditure may actually be lower, in relative terms, during exercise than at rest (Table 4). These data are entirely consistent with the notion that carbohydrates and fats are the major contributors to the rise in oxidative catabolism associated with exercise, as discussed above. However, the absolute rise in leucine oxidation during the 2 hr bicycle ergometer ride in our experiments equals 90% of the currently estimated daily leucine requirement. If the change in leucine oxidation is reflective of changes in the oxidation of other amino acids, it raises important questions regarding the leucine and total protein requirement in the diet of exercising individuals. Therefore, a somewhat more extensive account of the relationships between branched-chain amino acids, muscle amino acid metabolism, and exercise will be presented in the following section.

Body Metabolism of Amino Acids During Exercise

An integrated, whole-body view of amino acid metabolism during exercise has been proposed by Felig, Wahren, et al[18,20,40] (Table 5). Using arteriovenous catheterization techniques, they showed that exercise promotes a release of alanine from muscle tissue which is proportional to the intensity of the exercise performed. They further observed that an exercising limb selectively takes up branched-chain amino acids during prolonged exercise, while the splanchnic bed (gut and liver), on the other hand, releases equal amounts of the branched-chain amino acids and takes up increased amounts of alanine. On the basis of these findings and evidence from other investigators that muscle tissue preferentially catabolizes branched-chain amino acids, they propose that branched-chain amino acids may become important energy-yielding fuels during prolonged exercise, while at the same time providing nitrogen for alanine formation. It has been suggested by Felig, Wahren and colleagues[18,20,40] and others[41-43] that alanine serves as a vehicle for nitrogen transport from muscles to the liver, where it contributes its carbon skeleton for glucose production and its nitrogen to urea. The urea is then excreted through the sweat and urine. This scheme is attractive, since it explains both the increase in leucine oxidation and the increase in urea production which have been measured during prolonged exercise.

Other possibilities may be considered. The increase in branched-chain amino acid oxidation rate could provide energy either for contracting muscles or for meeting the increased metabolic demands of the liver during exercise. Earlier studies suggest that after leucine is transaminated in skeletal muscle, its α-keto acid diffuses out of the muscle and is transported to the liver, where it is oxidized. This scheme is partly based on analyses of *in vitro* enzyme activity, which suggest that skeletal muscle does not have a great capacity for the complete oxidation of branched-chain amino acids. However, the work of

Table 5. Arterial Concentration and Exchange of Amino Acids Across the Leg and Splanchnic Bed at the End of a 4 h Bicycle Exercise at ~30% VO_2 max*

Amino Acid	Arterial Concentration		Exchange		Leg	
	Rest	240 min Exercise	Splanchnic		Rest	240 min Exercise
			Rest	@240 min		
	—µmol/1—		—µmol/1—			
Glycine	188	160	8.3	31.8†	−8	17.8†
Alanine	192	233	57.6	119.0†	−30.4	−95.4†
Leucine	126	151†	−2.2	−30.2†	−0.8	28.6†
Valine	242	243	−3.2	−31.6†	−0.6	43.4†
Isoleucine	60	81†	−1.0	−17.2†	−0.4	21.8†

*Partial summary of data of Ahlborg et al.[20]
†Significantly different p < 0.05 from value at rest.
Reproduced with permission. See footnote on p. 51.

Odessey and Goldberg[44] and others[13] indicates that muscle is capable of completely oxidizing these amino acids.

The view that muscle is capable of significant amino acid oxidation is supported by a consideration of the relative energy demands of muscle and liver. During exercise, the energy demand of skeletal muscle increases tremendously, and a greater than tenfold increase in oxygen consumption is not uncommon. While the energy demand of the liver also increases during prolonged exercise,[40] the increased energy expenditure by the liver may be only one-tenth of that in muscle. However, if the increased oxidation of amino acids during exercise does not occur in muscle, but in the liver, then using a conservative estimate of 5% contribution by amino acid oxidation to the whole-body energy demand, amino acid oxidation would account for more than 60% of the total energy demand of the liver. This seems unlikely, and it is thus reasonable to assume that the major site of enhanced amino acid catabolism during exercise is in the working muscles.

The oxidation of leucine in particular seems to be coordinately regulated with the oxidation of carbohydrate and fat substrates during exercise. The rate-limiting step in the oxidation of branched-chain amino acids in muscle is the decarboxylation step, and this occurs in the mitochondria.[45] The activity of branched-chain amino acid α-keto-dehydrogenase, the controlling enzyme, has been shown to be regulated by many of the products of leucine oxidation, including acetyl coenzyme A (CoA).[46] In this respect, its regulation is similar to that of pyruvate dehydrogenase. During exercise, the greatly increased flux of acetyl CoA through the citric acid cycle depletes the acetyl CoA pool.[13,40] This reduction in the acetyl CoA pool, along with changes in intracellular ATP and intramitochondrial nicotinamide adenine dinucleotide-reduced (NADH) levels, stimulates the flow of carbohydrates and free fatty acids through their respective degradative pathways and also stimulates the activity of the branched-chain amino acid α-keto-dehydrogenase,[46] thereby increasing the flow of leucine through its degradative pathway. This results in a loss of leucine and a generation of acetyl CoA.

One factor which may modify the extent to which leucine is oxidized is the intensity at which the exercise is performed. Millward and associates[39] have reported that the rate of whole body leucine oxidation increases with increasing exercise intensity. This further indicates that as the reliance on free fatty acid oxidation for energy decreases, the relative contribution of carbohydrate and branched-chain amino acid oxidation increases. However, because the catabolism of branched-chain amino acids is an oxidative process, an increasing reliance on glycolysis for energy at intensities above $\dot{V}O_2$ max would decrease amino acid oxidation rates. Hence, during sprint-type activities or weight-lifting, where anaerobic metabolism predominates, little protein oxidation would be expected.

Dietary Protein Requirement for Regularly Exercising Individuals

In the first section of this review we cited evidence which shows that regular exercise has a definite anabolic effect, promoting an increase in lean body mass; yet, in the second section, we cited evidence which shows that single episodes of moderate exercise result in increased catabolism of amino acids and increased losses of body nitrogen. Since both long-term anabolic and short-term catabolic effects obviously occur, the period following each episode of moderate exercise must be an especially anabolic period of protein metabolism, during which the conservation of endogenous amino acids and the utilization of dietary protein both improve. Adequate human studies of amino acid and whole body protein metabolism during this immediate post-exercise period have not been reported and should be conducted. If this post-exercise anabolic period response is inadequate, then the dietary intake of protein must increase to achieve an increase in lean body mass. A number of long-term nitrogen balance studies have addressed the question as to whether the dietary protein intake must be increased during periods of regular exercise to maintain nitrogen balance. These are summarized in Table 6 and are described in more detail below.

Gontzea et al[47] conducted a large, carefully-controlled study in which 30 healthy young men consumed a diet containing 1.0 g protein/kg body weight. Nitrogen balance determinations were done for three periods, a sedentary

Table 6. Nitrogen Balance Studies of Dietary Protein Requirements for Exercise

Investigators	Exercise Period	Protein Intake (g/kg·day)	Nitrogen Balance
Gontzea et al[47,48]	4 days	1.0	Negative
	4 days	1.5	Positive
	3 weeks	1.0	Initially negative, approached equilibrium after 2–3 weeks
Consolazio et al[49]	40 days	1.4	Positive
	40 days	2.4	More positive than for lower protein group
Marable et al[50]	28 days	0.8	Decrease in urinary N excretion during last 14 days for both groups when compared to controls.
	28 days	2.4	
Celejowa and Homa[51]	11 days	2.0	Slightly positive

Note: The type and intensity of exercise used in these studies are described in the text.

adaptation period, a four-day exercise period, and a four-day sedentary post-exercise period. The daily exercise consisted of six 20 minute intervals on a bicycle ergometer at a work effort of 8–10 kcal/min, separated by 30 minute breaks. Energy expenditure was re-examined during the exercise period and the total energy intake was increased accordingly to provide an average of 50 kcal/kg body weight per day. Sweat nitrogen losses were included in the calculation of nitrogen balance. The mean nitrogen balance became negative during the exercise period and did not become positive even when the dietary protein intake was increased to 1.5 g/kg body weight. In a second study, Gontzea et al[48] examined the effect of a longer training period on nitrogen balance using a similar exercise load and a diet containing 1.0 g protein/kg body weight. Nitrogen balance became negative with the onset of the exercise period but approached equilibrium by 2 weeks of training (Fig 3).

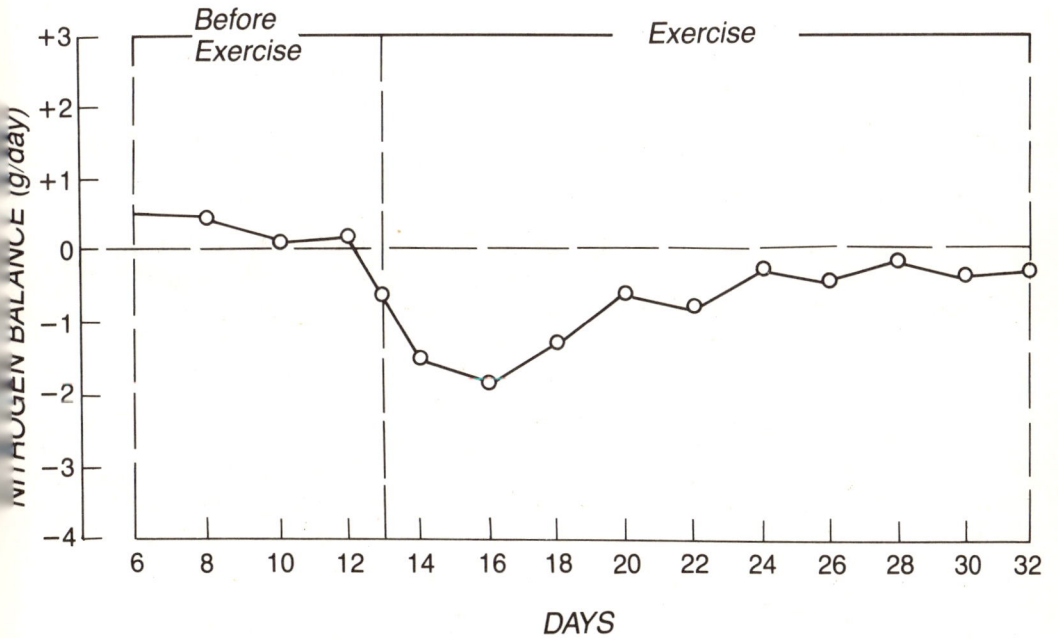

From: GONTZEA et al (1975)

Figure 3. Mean nitrogen balance for 12 healthy young men before and during a 3-week period of increased physical activity (exercise energy expenditure was 9.9 kcal/min for six 20 min periods per day). Subjects received 1 g protein/kg body weight per day (35% from animal origin). Drawn from Gontzea et al.[48] Reproduced with permission. See footnote on page 50.

Consolazio et al[49] studied subjects consuming 1.4 or 2.8 g protein/kg body weight per day and 3700 kcal energy per day. The exercise regimen was varied and lasted 40 days. Sweat nitrogen losses were measured. Both groups were in positive nitrogen balance throughout the study, although the balances were more strikingly positive for subjects consuming the higher protein diet.

Marable et al[50] placed untrained college men on a progressive weight training program. Control and exercise groups consumed the Recommended Dietary Allowance (RDA) for protein (0.8 g/kg body weight per day)[1] during one period and 3 times this level (2.4 g/kg body weight per day) during the other. Energy was provided in amounts which produced a small deliberate weight gain in all subjects, except in those subjects in the control group consuming the RDA for protein, who lost weight. Exercising groups gained a mean 3.2 kg during the 28 days of the study while receiving a mean of 62 kcal energy/kg body weight per day. Only urinary nitrogen was analyzed, and exercising groups excreted less nitrogen than their controls. However, it should be noted that the weight gain was more positive in the exercising subjects, and it is impossible to judge whether the reduction in nitrogen output was due to the exercise or to a surfeit of energy.

Ten Polish weight lifters training for the Olympics were studied by Celejowa and Homa.[51] Subjects consumed an average of 2 g protein/kg body weight and 50 kcal energy/kg body weight per day. Daily training energy expenditure for both weight lifting and general conditioning exercises was about 1500 kcal. Sweat nitrogen losses were measured and included in the nitrogen balance calculations. Although nitrogen balance was, on the average, slightly positive, five subjects were in negative nitrogen balance for the 11 days of the study.

Torun et al[52] measured both nitrogen balance and total body potassium in college students participating in an isometric exercise program. Protein was provided at 0.5 or 1.0 g/kg body weight per day and energy was supplied at a level sufficient to maintain body weight (45–55 kcal/kg body weight per day). Although nitrogen balance data were not consistent, exercising subjects consuming the lower level of protein lost body potassium, suggesting that body cell mass could not be maintained at this level of protein intake.

The conclusion which must be drawn is that exercising individuals have difficulty maintaining nitrogen balance when the dietary protein is provided at a level less than about 1.0–1.5 g/kg body weight per day. Several lines of evidence imply, therefore, that the requirement for total protein and certain indispensable amino acids is higher for individuals exercising regularly at moderate to heavy intensities. This appears to be particularly true for individuals undergoing a training program. On the other hand, we do not find sufficient evidence to support the intakes of up to 2.5 or 3.0 g/kg body weight per day which have been recommended by some authors.[53,54] We realize, however, that in practice, individuals participating in high-resistance weight training for increases in strength and muscle size regularly consume these high levels of protein.

Summary and Conclusions

Submaximal exercise results in greatly increased rates of indispensable amino acid oxidation coupled with increased urinary and sweat nitrogen excretion. This leads us to believe that current recommendations for minimum protein requirements may not be adequate for exercising individuals. This contrasts with the prevailing view that physical activity *per se* does not result in an increased need for dietary protein. Higher levels of protein intake may be of particular importance for those undertaking a program of aerobic exercise training, although their precise requirements have yet to be determined. The standard American diet, which provides protein in excess of 1 g/kg body weight per day, should be adequate for their protein needs. Protein needs for those undergoing a program of high-resistance weight training for increases in strength and muscle size are also unknown.

References

1. Food and Nutrition Board: *Recommended Dietary Allowances*, ed 9, National Academy of Sciences, National Research Council, Washington, 1980, pp 39–54.
2. Food and Agriculture Organization/World Health Organization: *Energy and Protein Requirements*, Tech Rep Ser No 522, Geneva, 1973, pp 1–118.
3. Young VR: Skeletal muscle and whole body protein metabolism in relation to exercise, in Poortmans J, Niset G (eds): *Biochemistry of Exercise: Exercise and Hormone Regulations*. Baltimore, University Park Press, 1981, pp 59–74.
4. Young VR, Munro HN: N^T-methylhistidine (3-methylhistidine) and muscle protein turnover: an overview. *Fed Proc* 37:2291–2300, 1978.
5. Young VR: The role of skeletal and cardiac muscle in the regulation of protein metabolism, in Munro HN (ed): *Mammalian Protein Metabolism*. New York, Academic Press, 1970, pp 585–674.
6. Gollnick PD, Armstrong RB, Saubert CW, et al: Enzyme activity and fiber composition in skeletal muscle of untrained and trained men. *J Appl Physiol* 33:321–323, 1972.
7. Saltin B: Metabolic fundamentals in exercise. *Med Sci Sports* 5:137–146, 1973.
8. Holloszy JO, Booth FW: Biochemical adaptations to endurance exercise in muscle. *Ann Rev Physiol* 56:273–291, 1976.
9. Costill DL, Fink WJ, Pollack ML: Muscle fiber composition and enzyme activities of elite distance runners. *Med Sci Sports* 8:96–100, 1976.
10. Goldberg Al, Etlinger JD, Goldspink DF, et al: Mechanisms of work-induced hypertrophy of skeletal muscle. *Med Sci Sports* 7:185–198, 1975.
11. Laurent GJ, Sparrow MP: Changes in RNA, DNA and protein content and the rates of protein synthesis and degradation during hypertrophy of the anterior latissimus dorsi muscle of the adult fowl (Gallus Domesticus). *Growth* 41:249–262, 1977.
12. Laurent GJ, Sparrow MP, Millward DJ: Turnover of muscle protein in the fowl. Changes in rates of protein synthesis and breakdown during hypertrophy of the anterior and posterior latissimus dorsi muscles. *Biochem J* 176:407–417, 1978.
13. Saltin B, Karlsson J: Muscle glycogen utilization during work of different intensities, in Pernow B, Saltin B (eds): *Muscle Metabolism During Exercise*, ed 11. New York, Plenum Press, 1971, pp 289–300.
14. Costill DL, Sparks KE, Gregor R, et al: Muscle glycogen utilization during exhaustion running. *J Appl Physiol* 31:353–356, 1971.
15. Costill DL, Thomason H, Roberts E: Fractional utilization of the aerobic capacity during distance running. *Med Sci Sports* 5:248–252, 1973.
16. Bessman SP, Geiger PJ: Transport of energy in muscle: the phosphorylcreatine shuttle. *Science* 211:448–452, 1981.
17. Åstrand PO: Nutrition and physical performance, in *Nutrition and the World Food Problem*. Basel, Karger Press, 1979, p 63.
18. Felig P, Wahren J: Fuel homeostasis in exercise. *N Engl J Med* 293:1078–1084, 1975.
19. di Prompero PE: Energetics of muscular exercise. *Rev Physiol Biochem Pharmacol* 89:143–222, 1981.
20. Ahlborg G, Felig P, Hagenfeldt L, et al: Substrate turnover during prolonged exercise in man. Splanchnic and leg metabolism of glucose, free fatty acids, and amino acids. *J Clin Invest* 53:1080–1090, 1974.

21. Lemon PWR, Nagle FJ: Effects of exercise on protein and amino acid metabolism. *Med Sci Sport Exerc* 13:141–149, 1981.

22. Phinney SD, Bistrian BR, Evans WJ, et al: The human metabolic response to chronic ketosis without caloric restriction: preservation of submaximal exercise capability with reduced carbohydrate oxidation. *Metabolism* (in press), 1982.

23. von Liebig J: Die Quelle der Muskelkraft. *Ann Chemie Pharmacie* 153:157–228, 1870.

24. Fick A, Wisclicenus J: On the origin of muscular power. *Philosophical Magazine and Journal of Science* 31:485–503, 1866.

25. Cathcart EP: The influence of muscle work on protein metabolism. *Physiol Rev* 5:225–243, 1925.

26. Décombaz J, Reinhardt P, Anantharaman K, et al: Biochemical changes in a 100 km run: free amino acids, urea and creatinine. *Eur J Appl Physiol* 41:61–72, 1979.

27. Refsum HE, Strömme SB: Urea and creatinine excretion in urine during and after prolonged heavy exercise. *Scand J Clin Lab Invest* 33:247–254, 1974.

28. Haralambie G, Berg A: Serum urea and amino nitrogen changes with exercise duration. *Europ J Appl Physiol* 36:39–48, 1976.

29. Cerny F: Protein metabolism during two hour ergometer exercise, in Howald J, Poortmans JR (eds): *Metabolic adaptation to prolonged physical exercise*. Basel, Birkhäuser Verlag, 1973, pp 232–237.

30. Calloway DH, Odell ACF, Margen S: Sweat and miscellaneous nitrogen losses in human balance studies. *J Nutr* 101:775–786, 1971.

31. Lemon PWR, Mullin JP: Effect of initial muscle glycogen levels on protein catabolism during exercise. *J Appl Physiol: Respirat Environ Exercise Physiol* 48:624–629, 1980.

32. Poortmans JR: Effects of long lasting physical exercise and training on protein metabolism, in Howald H Poortmans JR (eds): *Metabolic adaptation to prolonged physical exercise*. Basel, Birkhäuser Verlag, 1973, pp 212–225.

33. Brodan V, Kuhn E, Pechar J, et al: Changes of free amino acids in plasma of healthy subjects induced by physical exercise. *Europ J Appl Physiol* 35:69–77, 1976.

34. Dohm GL, Hecker AL, Brown WE, et al: Adaptation of protein metabolism to endurance training: increased amino acid oxidation in response to training. *Biochem J* 164:705–708, 1977.

35. Young VR, Bier DM: Stable isotopes (^{13}C and ^{15}N) in the study of human protein and amino acid metabolism and requirements; in Beers RF, Bassett EG (eds): *Nutritional Factors: Modulating Effects on Metabolic Processes*. New York, Raven Press, 1981, pp 267–308.

36. Waterlow JC: Lysine turnover in man measured by intravenous infusion of L-[U-^{14}C]lysine. *Clin Sci* 33:507–515, 1967.

37. Waterlow JC, Garlick PJ, Millward DJ: *Protein Turnover in Mammalian Tissues and in the Whole Body*. New York, Elsevier/North Holland, 1978, pp 1–804.

38. Rennie MJ, Halliday D, Davies CTM, et al: Exercise induced increase in leucine oxidation in man and the effect of glucose, in Walser M, William JR (eds): *Metabolism and Clinical Implications of Branched Chain Amino and Keto-acids*. New York, Elsevier/North Holland, 1981, pp 361–366.

39. Millward DJ, Davies CTM, Halliday D, et al: The effect of exercise on protein metabolism in man as explored with stable isotopes. *Fed Proc* 1981, (In press).

40. Felig P, Wahren J: Amino acid metabolism in exercising man. *J Clin Invest* 50:2703–2714, 1971.

41. Chochinov RH, Perlman K, Moorhouse JA: Circulating alanine production and disposal in healthy subjects. *Diabetes* 27:287–295, 1978.

42. Lund P: Precursors of urea synthesis, in Waterlow JC, Stephen JML (eds): *Nitrogen Metabolism in Man*. London, Applied Science Publishers, 1981, pp 197–202.

43. Goldberg AL, Chang TW: Regulation and significance of amino acid metabolism in skeletal muscle. *Fed Proc* 37:2301–2307, 1978.

44. Odessey R, Goldberg AL: Oxidation of leucine by rat skeletal muscle. *Am J Physiol* 223:1376–1383, 1972.

45. Danner DJ, Sewell ET, Elsas LJ: Regulation of solubilized branched chain ketoacid dehydrogenase complex, in Walser EM, Williamson JR (eds): *Metabolism and Clinical Implications of Branched Chain Amino and Ketoacids*. New York, Elsevier/North-Holland, 1981, pp 29–34.

46. Williamson JR, Martin-Requero A, Corkey BE, et al: Interactions of α-ketoisovalerate, propionate and fatty acids on gluconeogenesis and ureagenesis in isolated hepatocytes, in Walser EM, Williamson JR (eds): *Metabolism and Clinical Implications of Branched Chain Amino and Ketoacids*. New York, Elsevier/North-Holland, 1981, pp 105–109.

47. Gontzea I, Sutzescu P, Dumitrache S: The influence of muscular activity on nitrogen balance and on the need of man for proteins. *Nutrition Reports International* 10:35–43, 1974.

48. Gontzea I, Sutzescu R, Dumitrache S: The influence of adaptation to physical effort on nitrogen balance in man. *Nutrition Reports International* 11:231–236, 1975.

49. Consolazio CF, Johnson HL, Nelson RA, et al: Protein metabolism during intensive physical training in the young adult. *Am J Clin Nutr* 28:29–35, 1975.

50. Marable NL, Hickson Jr JF, Korslund MK, et al: Urinary nitrogen excretion as influenced by a muscle-building exercise program and protein intake variation. *Nutrition Reports International* 19:795–805, 1979.

51. Celejowa I, Homa M: Food intake, nitrogen and energy balance in Polish weight lifters, during a training camp. *Nutr Metab* 12:259–274, 1970.

52. Torun B, Scrimshaw NS, Young VR: Effect of isometric exercises on body potassium and dietary protein requirements of young men. *Am J Clin Nutr* 30:1983–1993, 1977.

53. Strauzenberg SE, Schneider F, Donath R, et al: The problem of dieting in training and athletic performance. *Biblthca Nutr Dieta:* 27:133–142, 1979.

54. Ryan AJ: Anabolic steroids are fool's gold. *Fed Proc* 40:2682–2688, 1981.

INTERRELATION OF PHYSICAL ACTIVITY AND NUTRITION ON BLOOD PRESSURE/CIRCULATION

Richard M. Schieken, MD*

Introduction

The disease "hypertension" is defined arbitrarily by the upper portion of the distribution of systolic or diastolic blood pressure measurements. Using a working definition that lacks information about the pathogenesis will most likely invoke confusion about causality. The purpose of this discussion is to explore the possible contributions of nutrition and physical exercise to the development or treatment of hypertension. The evidence that either nutritional or physical exertion abnormalities are causal or therapeutic is meager. Two major factors frequently implicated in both pathogenesis and treatment of hypertension are sodium and obesity. While physical exercise has been claimed to decrease blood pressure, the mechanism of this effect is unclear.

This chapter will provide an overview of the relationship of sodium, obesity, and physical exercise to the development and treatment of hypertension.

Sodium

In any discussion of the mechanisms responsible for hypertension, dietary sodium intake is inexorably linked as an etiologic agent. Historically, western man has used salt as a condiment, eating salt well beyond his physiologic need.[1] The word "salary" has its root from the latin word "salarium" meaning salt money, which the Romans paid their soldiers. Some people would argue that the punishment for man's greed for salt is hypertension.

Though hypertension and its attendant morbidity can be induced in animals by abnormal diet or selective breeding,[2,3] spontaneous hypertension is apparently a unique human condition which does not appear to occur in free living animals in nature.

For many years, investigators have suspected a relationship between dietary intake of sodium and hypertension. The evidence for this association is based upon 1) epidemiologic studies of unacculturated populations who, on the average, ingest small amounts of sodium and, coincidentally, maintain low average population blood pressures, 2) clinical observations of the effect of sodium reduction in ameliorating preexisting hypertension and, 3) animal experiments linking high sodium intake to experimental hypertension and stroke in genetically predisposed animals.

---

*The University of Iowa Hospitals and Clinics, Iowa City, Iowa

Epidemiologic Studies

Many widely separated populations who are not acculturated to western social patterns not only do not develop hypertension, but also do not demonstrate an increase in blood pressure with age.[4] Despite a presumably wide variation in dietary patterns from population to population, common to most of these societies is the fact that their average dietary sodium intake was well below that of western people (Table 1).

Table 1. Sodium intake of low blood-pressure populations

Society	Sodium (mEq/24 hr)
Yanomama Indians, Brazil	±1.5
Tukisenta, New Guinea	±15
Kwaio, Baegu, Aita, Solomon Islands	10–20
Pukapuka, Cook Islands	±65
Samburur, Uganda	±50
Ontong Java, Solomon Islands	50–70

Reprinted with permission from Page LB[7] (Courtesy of Raven Press)

Though the studies of these populations purport to show a strong correlation between low sodium intake and the generally low level of blood pressure, an analysis of the dominant effects of acculturation *per se* was neglected. A study of the people of the Solomon Islands[5] grouped the societies according to the degree of their western acculturation. In this study, some evidence was provided for the association of blood pressure and body weight. Investigators find that body weight is a major confounding variable when they study the relationship of diet to blood pressure in studies of large populations. Moreover, as western acculturation increases in a society, so also does crowding, alcohol intake, urban living, noise, and varied socioeconomic status. The relationship of physical activity to the changes that occur with western acculturation have not been completely studied.

Nonetheless, despite the argument of the presence of these many confounding variables as possible contributors to hypertension in western populations, a study of the Qash'qai people (relatively isolated mountain nomads living in southern Iran) who eat large amounts of salt, shows that despite their lean habitus, hard work and traditional lifestyle, hypertension is found in about 15% of the total population.[6] Increases in blood pressure with age in male Qash'qai are positively correlated with sodium excretion; among females, increases in blood pressure with age are positively correlated with the sodium to potassium ratio (Na/K). Moreover, the Qash'qai diet is relatively potassium poor with Na/K ratios of approximately 3.5, based on analytic dietary data.

Though many factors affect blood pressure, sodium intake is a powerful determinant. A somewhat puzzling pattern emerges, however, from the popula-

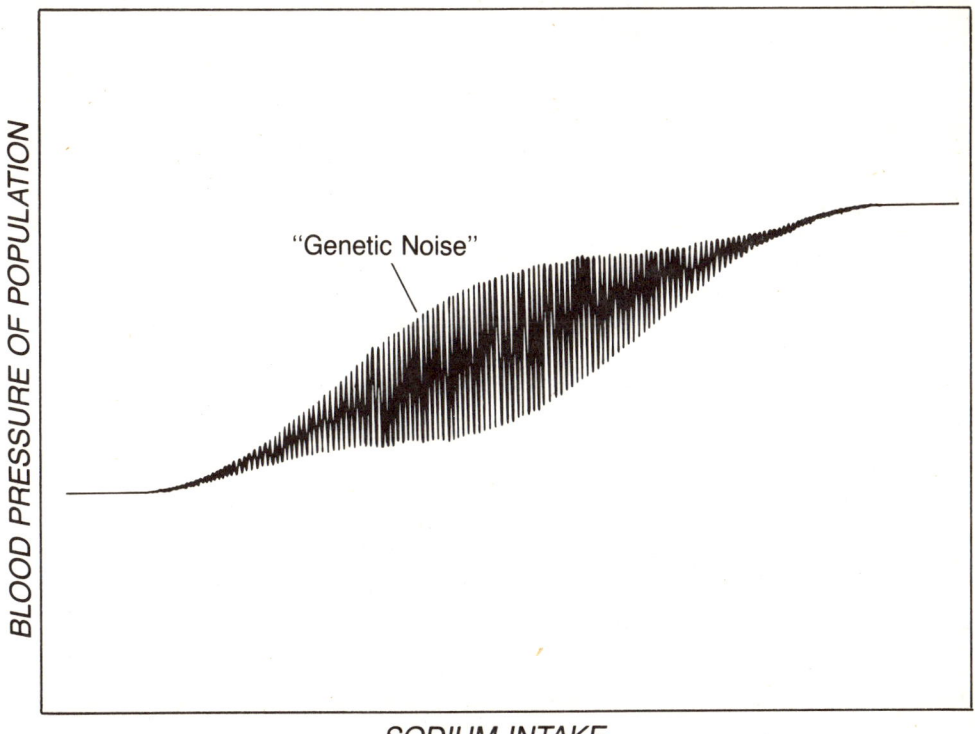

Figure 1. Probable relationship of sodium intake and blood pressure in populations. Reprinted with permission from Page LB[7]. (Courtesy of Raven Press).

tion studies. Page has summarized the evidence as illustrated in Figure 1. When all individuals in a population habitually ingest small amounts of sodium, the average blood pressure is low and does not increase with age. On the other hand, with average ingestion of large amounts of sodium, a high percentage of the population develops hypertension. Between these two extremes, Page describes a wide variability in the relationship between blood pressure and sodium intake caused by variable genetic susceptibility and other major confounders present in society.

Clinical Studies

Early clinical studies by Ambard and Beaujard[8] and Allen and Sherill[9] demonstrated that a diet extremely low in sodium could reduce blood pressure in hypertensive individuals. Later, Kempner popularized the rice-fruit diet, one of the first organized attempts to treat hypertension by extreme dietary restriction of sodium.[10] Those studies have shown that a diet low to extremely low in sodium could ameliorate existing hypertension;[11] reintroduction of sodium into the diets of these individuals raises the blood pressure. This effect is not seen in all individuals.[12] Salt restriction can be used to reduce the blood pressure in some patients. However, compliance is not very good.[13] Experimental studies in rats demonstrate that the addition of potassium chloride to a diet high in sodium chloride provides some protection against the morbidity of high blood pressure.[14] Sasaki et al showed a similar protective effect in patients.[15]

In cultures such as that of the United States, in which the use of prepared foods containing considerable sodium is widespread, Dustan et al claimed that very low sodium diets have little place in the treatment of hypertension when renal function is sufficient to allow diuretic drugs to have an effect.[16] Common clinical practice today is to advise both diuretic therapy and a moderate reduction in dietary sodium intake to levels of 5 gm of sodium chloride per day (2,000 mg).[17]

Experimental Hypertension

Through selective breeding, laboratory rats have been developed that are either hypertension-prone or hypertension-resistant.[18] When ingesting a low sodium diet, neither strain of rat becomes hypertensive. As salt is added to their diet to a level of 8% sodium chloride, the susceptible rats become increasingly hypertensive.

Guyton et al have suggested a possible pathogenic mechanism linking sodium ingestion to an increase in extracellular fluid volume.[19] He observed that after a salt and water loading, there was a temporary rise in cardiac output followed by an elevated peripheral vascular resistance. The next step in the sequence is an increase in urinary output resulting in a reduction in extracellular fluid volume. From these observations, Guyton et al designed a systems analysis flow diagram to illustrate the interrelationship of the various "feedback loops" involved in the regulation of blood pressure.

In summary, epidemiologic, clinical and experimental findings show that sodium intake appears to be an important, but not singular determinant of blood pressure. Unacculturated populations who eat lower average amounts of salt rarely develop hypertension. Potassium may exert a protective effect. Lowering the amount of salt ingested by hypertensive patients to approximately 5 gm per day (2000 mg sodium) appears to be safe and may reduce blood pressure in some individuals. In the medical management of hypertensive patients, salt reduction frequently enhances the antihypertensive effect of diuretics.[17]

Obesity

In many studies, weight and blood pressure are positively correlated. Thus people who weigh more have higher blood pressure. The Framingham Study[20] showed that the average blood pressure level increased as relative weight increased. However, the correlation between relative weight (weight compared to median weight of the cohort of the same height and expressed as a percentage over or under the standard "weight" set as 100) with systolic blood pressure was modest (r = 0.3). Systolic blood pressure also correlated with measures of adiposity such as triceps skinfold thickness and upper arm girth. The Framingham Study also described the risk of developing hypertension in normotensive obese individuals or normotensives who later gain appreciable amounts of weight.

In the Evans County Study,[21] similar associations were observed. The investigators also stated that despite the high correlation that exists between excess body weight and hypertension, when hypertension occurs in lean men, there is an even stronger association with the development of coronary heart disease.

In studies involving the school children of Muscatine, Iowa, the prevalence of elevated blood pressure was high among overweight children (weight above the 90th percentile for height and age).[22] Twenty-seven percent of the overweight children had systolic blood pressure and twenty-four percent had diastolic blood pressure above the 90th percentile.

Reisin et al[23] studied the effect of weight loss without salt restriction on the reduction of blood pressure in overweight hypertensive patients. All patients lost weight and decreased their blood pressure. The weight and blood pressure reduction were significant in both sexes and all ages and were directly related one to another.

In summary, there is ample evidence that weight is positively correlated with blood pressure and that loss of weight, independent of salt intake, will reduce blood pressure.

Physical Exercise

Millions of healthy Americans participate in strenuous athletic activities. Recently Carr et al[24] showed that chronic exercise training in young women increased plasma levels of Beta-Endorphin, a naturally occurring opioid-peptide. Thus, chronic exercise induces a "natural high". Aside from feeling good from our natural opioid-peptides, whether or not exercise treats hypertension is controversial.

Johnson and Grover showed no reduction of blood pressure in four hypertensive subjects submitted to a conditioning program of four weeks duration.[25] Most studies on the effects of exercise on the blood pressure of young subjects during training have shown small and insignificant changes.[26,27]

The response to exercise is different in individuals with elevated blood pressure. In adults, during invasive studies, Levy et al found that the calculated peripheral vascular resistance was both significantly higher at rest and during graded treadmill exercise in hypertensives.[28] Amery et al had similar observations adding that maximal voluntary oxygen consumption and cardiac output were significantly reduced with increasing severity of hypertension.[29] They also noted a decline in oxygen consumption and cardiac output and an increase in systolic blood pressure with age.

James found that children with elevated resting systolic blood pressure achieved significantly higher exercise systolic blood pressure than normotensive controls.[30] Our data, across the normal distribution of children's systolic blood pressure, are similar. We found that children with persistently elevated resting blood pressures continue to have significantly higher blood pressures during exercise (Figure 2). The resting cardiac output correlates with blood pressure and cardiac output during isometric exercise. Therefore, the dominant resting hemodynamic determinant of resting blood pressure (cardiac output or systemic vascular resistance) continues to be the dominant determinant during exercise.[31]

Middle-aged men who participated in a vigorous training program had significant reductions in both systolic blood pressure and diastolic blood pressure without weight loss.[32] Boyer and Kasch reported similar findings in patients with more severe hypertension who required continued antihypertensive therapy. However, the data were not adjusted for weight loss.[33]

Exercise programs appear to be a valuable adjunct in the therapy of hypertension. After careful screening for coronary risk, blood pressure can be reduced through a supervised program which includes gradually increasing levels of exercise, weight loss (when appropriate), moderate sodium restriction and pharmacologic agents.

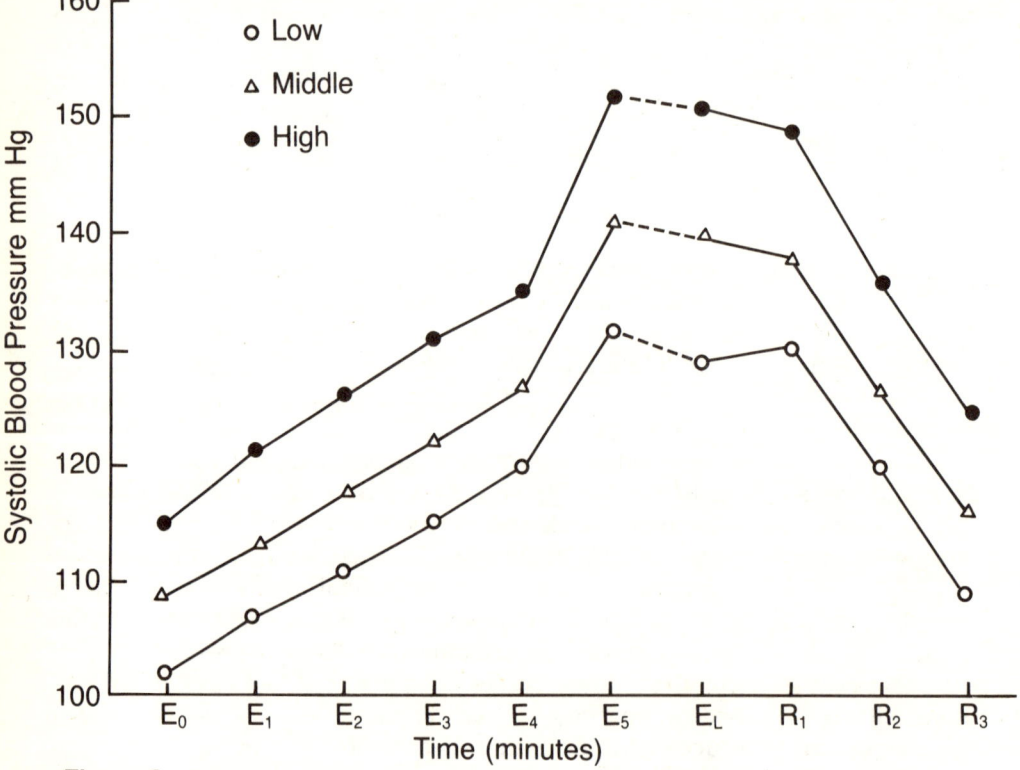

Figure 2. Children in the highest, middle and lowest quintiles of resting systolic blood pressure maintain significant systolic blood pressure differences throughout dynamic exercise and recovery.

References

1. Meneely GR, Battarbee HG: High sodium low potassium environment and hypertension. *Am J Cardiol* 38:768–784, 1976.
2. Dahl LK: Effects of chronic excess salt feeding: Induction of self-sustaining hypertension in rats. *J Exp Med* 114:231–236, 1961.
3. Okamoto KA, Aoki K: Development of a strain of spontaneously hypertensive rats. *Japanese Circulation Journal* 27:282–293, 1963.
4. Meneely GR, Dahl LK: Electrolytes in hypertension: The effects of sodium chloride. *Med Clin North Am* 45:271–283, 1961.
5. Page LB, Damor A, Moellering RC: Antecedents of cardiovascular disease in six Solomon Islands societies. *Circulation* 49:1132–1146, 1974.
6. Page LB, Vandevert D, Nader K, et al: Blood pressure, diet, and body form in traditional nomads of the Qash'qai tribe, Southern Iran. *Acta Cardiol* 33:102–103, 1978.
7. Page LB: Dietary sodium and blood pressure: Evidence from human studies, in Lauer RM, Shekelle RB (eds): *Childhood Prevention of Atherosclerosis and Hypertension*. New York, Raven Press, 1980, pp 291–303.
8. Ambard L, Beaujard E: Causes de l'hypertension and arterielle. *Arch Gen Med* 1:520–533, 1904.
9. Allen FM, Sherill JW: The treatment of arterial hypertension. *J Metab Res* 2:429–545, 1922.
10. Kempner W: Treatment of hypertensive vascular disease with rice diet. *Am J Med* 4:545–577, 1948.
11. Perera G, Blood DW: The relationship of sodium chloride to hypertension. *J Clin Invest* 26:1109–1118, 1947.
12. Brown WJ, Brown K, Krishian I: Exchangeable sodium and blood volume in normotensive and hypertensive humans on high and low sodium intake. *Circulation* 43:508–519, 1971.
13. Morgan T, Adam W, Gillies A, et al: Hypertension treated by salt restriction. *Lancet* 1:227, 1978.
14. Meneely GR, Ball COT, Youmans JB: Chronic sodium chloride toxicity: The protective effect of added potassium chloride. *Ann Intern Med* 47:263–273, 1957.
15. Sasaki N, Mitsuhashi T, Fukushi S: The effects of the ingestion of large amounts of apples on blood pressure in farmers in Aquita prefercture. *Igaku To Seidutsugaku* 51:103–105, 1959.
16. Dustan HR, Tarazi C, Bravo EL: Diuretic and diuril treatment of hypertension. *Arch Intern Med* 133:1007–1013, 1974.
17. Parijs J, Joossens JV, Van der Linden L, et al: Moderate sodium restriction and diuretics in the treatment of hypertension. *Am Hrt J* 85:22–34, 1973.
18. Dahl LK: Salt and hypertension. *Am J Clin Nutr* 25:231–244, 1972.
19. Guyton AC, Coleman TG, Cowley AW, et al: A systems analysis approach to understanding long-range arterial blood pressure control and hypertension. *Circ Res* 35:159–176, 1974.
20. Kannel WB, Brand N, Skinner JJ, et al: The relation of adiposity to blood pressure and development of hypertension. The Framingham study. *Ann Intern Med* 67:48–59, 1967.
21. Tyroler HA, Heyden S, Bartel A, et al: Blood pressure and cholesterol as coronary heart disease risk factors. *Arch Intern Med* 128:907–914, 1971.

22. Lauer RM, Connor WE, Leaverton PE, et al: Coronary heart disease risk factors in school children: The Muscatine Study. *J Pediatr* 86:697–706, 1975.

23. Reisin E, Abel R, Modan M, et al: Effect of weight loss without salt restriction on the reduction of blood pressure in overweight hypertensive patients. *N Engl J Med* 298:1–6, 1978.

24. Carr DB, Bullen BA, Skrina GS, et al: Physical conditioning facilitates the exercise induced secretion of beta-endorphin an beta-litotropine. *N Eng J Med* 305:560–562, 1981.

25. Johnson WP, Grover JA: Hemodynamic and metabolic effects of physical training in four patients with essential hypertension. *Can Med Assoc J* 96:842, 1967.

26. Ekblom B, Astrand P, Saltin B, et al: Effect of training on circulatory response to exercise. *J Appl Physiol* 24:518, 1968.

27. Frick MH, Konttinen A, Sarajas HSS: Effects of physical training on circulation at rest and during exercise. *Am J Cardiol* 12:142, 1963.

28. Levy AM, Tabakin BS, Hanson JS: Hemodynamic responses to graded treadmill exercise in young untreated labile hypertensive patients. *Circulation* 35:1063–1072, 1967.

29. Amery A, Julius S, Witlock LS, et al: Influence of hypertension on the hemodynamic response to exercise. *Circulation* 36:231–237, 1967.

30. James FW: Effects of physical stress on adolescents with normal or abnormal cardiovascular function. *Post Grad Med* 56:53, 1974.

31. Schieken R, Clarke W, Lauer R: The cardiovascular responses to exercise in children across the blood pressure distribution: The Muscatine study. *Hypertension*, in press.

32. Choquette G, Ferguson RJ: Blood pressure reduction in borderline hypertensives following physical training. *Can Med Assoc J* 108:699–703, 1973.

33. Boyer JL, Kasch FW: Exercise therapy in hypertensive men. *JAMA* 211:1668–1671, 1970.

SOME INFLUENCES ON LEAN BODY MASS: EXERCISE, ANDROGENS, PREGNANCY, AND FOOD

Gilbert B. Forbes, MD*

The fact that body fat in man is subject to various influences has been established; however, the factors (apart from age and sex) that govern the size of the lean component of body weight have received relatively little attention. Males have a larger lean body mass (LBM) than females from early adolescence on, and LBM has been shown to be a function of stature.[1] The obese of both sexes tend to have a large LBM,[2,3] and body nitrogen is lost during caloric deprivation. Athletes tend to have a larger LBM than sedentary persons,[3,4] which suggests the possibility that exercise and/or physical training may affect the size of the lean component of body weight. It is generally conceded that exercise and training can improve strength, endurance, and maximum oxygen consumption, and some investigators have documented a reduction in body fat.[3,5,6]

We have recently had the opportunity of recording the effects of exercise, of androgen administration, and of obesity and anorexia on the LBM. In addition, we have measured LBM in a number of pregnant women both early and late in pregnancy. These results, together with data published by others, are sufficient to permit an examination of the influence of several factors on LBM in man.

Subjects and Methods

Four groups of young adult subjects were studied prior to and subsequent to various exercise regimes. Group I consisted of 11 males and 4 female college students (non-athletes) who exercised for 10 to 58 hours over periods of 20 to 150 days. Each kept a diary of activities, which included jogging, running, bicycling, swimming, weight lifting, and various intramural sports. Group II consisted of one male and two female students who exercised vigorously and regularly for 46 to 61 days, with total exercise time of 68 to 240 hours. One student rode his bicycle across the U.S.A. (from east to west), averaging 85 miles (6.1 hours) for each of 41 days of a 61 day journey.[7] He kept a dietary record, and his calculated caloric intake while bicycling averaged 3200 calories more than his usual pre-exercise intake. A second student engaged in swimming, running, and calisthenics almost daily for a total of 124 hours during a 46 day period. The third subject instituted a program of bicycling, squash, and softball, totaling 68 hours within a period of 54 days. Each kept a diary of his/her activities.

---

*University of Rochester Medical Center, Rochester, New York

Group III consisted of 19 West Point football players who performed three times weekly on the Nautilus machine for six weeks in addition to their regular spring football training. Each session on the Nautilus machine lasted for one-half hour or to point of exhaustion, and was conducted under the supervision of Dr. James Peterson of the Physical Education Department at West Point. The subjects travelled to Rochester for the ^{40}K assays.

Group IV consisted of two professional athletes (a weight lifter and a "body builder"). After a slack period of five months, they trained vigorously and took large doses of androgens (self-prescribed) for seven months in preparation for a contest. The training was intense, and consisted of running in place, push-ups, weight-lifting, arm and leg flexion and extension against resistance for 20 hours each week; both exercised to the point of fatigue, and both complained of aches and muscle soreness. Various androgens were taken, either together or in sequence, in gradually increasing amounts* during the seven month training period. Protein and amino acid supplements and a high caloric diet were also a part of the regimen.

Data were also obtained on 50 white pregnant women, 16 to 30 years of age, each of whom had ^{40}K assays early in pregnancy and again late in pregnancy. Gain in LBM and total weight for the entire pregnancy was estimated from these two assays, under the assumption that appreciable gains did not occur prior to the 12th week. All pregnancies were considered normal, and were carried to full term.

Finally, we made ^{40}K assays on 23 female patients with established obesity and on ten patients with anorexia nervosa; body composition in these two groups was compared to that of 308 adolescent girls and women who were considered to be of normal weight.

Lean body mass was estimated by potassium-40 counting,[8] skinfold thickness with the Harpenden caliper, grip strength with a hand dynamometer, and stature with the Holtain stadiometer. Replicate assays of LBM in our whole body scintillation counter yield coefficients of variation of 2% to 3%. Several of the subjects had duplicate or triplicate assays of LBM, skinfold thickness, and body circumferences both prior to and at the completion of the exercise period. Arm muscle-bone circumference (AMBC) was calculated from arm circumference (AC) at mid-point of the upper arm and the average of biceps and triceps skinfolds, using the following formula: $AMBC(cm) = AC(cm) - \frac{\pi}{20}(T + B)$, where T and B stand for triceps and biceps skinfold thickness in millimeters. Except for the cross-country bicycle rider (Group II) who monitored his diet at 3100 calories before and after his journey, and at 6300 calories during his trip, diets were not recorded.

---

*Oxandrolone, stanozol, methandrostenolone, and nandrolone were taken orally, and testosterone cyclopentylpropionate and Primabolin (a product made in Italy, not available in the U.S.A.) were administered intramuscularly. The maximum amounts were 190 mg daily and 900 mg daily (as testosterone equivalents), respectively, for the weight lifter and the "body builder."

Results

Results for the first three groups of exercising subjects are listed in Table 1. For Groups I and III the magnitude of the standard deviations indicate that the changes in body weight and LBM were not significantly different from zero. The maximum weight gain was 2.7 kg, the maximum loss 6.2 kg; the maximum gain in LBM was 4.8 kg, the maximum loss 5.1 kg. It is apparent that the amount of exercise engaged in did not serve to augment LBM, even in circumstances involving supervised use of the Nautilus machine.

Group II subjects, for whom exercise was prolonged and sustained, fared better; two of the three subjects showed an increase in LBM, but only one had a decrease in body fat. However, when all of the subjects in Groups I to III are rearranged in groups based on changes in body weight (Figure 1), there appears to be a tendency for weight and LBM to change in concert, ie, those who lost weight during the exercise period tended also to lose LBM, and those who gained weight tended to gain LBM.

Superimposed on the graph are two horizontal lines (dotted) indicating the variation in LBM to be expected when an individual is assayed in our counter on two occasions at an interval of several days. Data are available for two non-exercising adults: for one, the average difference between the first and second assay was -0.1 kg, s.d. 1.10($N = 21$); for the other, the average difference was -0.3 kg, s.d. 0.93 ($N = 13$). Since neither subject engaged in any unusual activities or sustained significant changes in body weight between each set of assays, the horizontal lines indicate the variability to be expected in the absence of exercise.

When large doses of androgens are superimposed on a vigorous training program, there is a striking rise in LBM and a decrease in body fat (Table 2, Figure 2), with parallel changes in arm muscle-bone circumference and skinfold thickness, respectively. The "body builder" also showed an increase in hand-grip. It is also of interest that both subjects tended to revert to their pre-training status when they stopped training and taking androgens.

Since the adult LBM contains about 33 g N/kg,[9] it is possible to calculate the increment in body N for these two subjects; this turns out to be 2.5 to 2.6 g/day, a value approximating that determined by the nitrogen balance technique for male subjects taking androgens for a week or two.[10]

During the past several years, a number of subjects with anorexia nervosa and with obesity have had ^{40}K assays in our laboratory. The data on body composition were compared with data obtained from large numbers of subjects considered to be of normal weight. This information can serve to illustrate the influence of nutrition on body composition. Table 3 presents data for female subjects aged 14 to 50 years, classified according to body fat content. The subjects labelled as "normal" were recruited during the course of several years and were divided into two groups on the basis of body fat content. The data in Table 3 demonstrate that under-nutrition serves to decrease LBM and that overnutrition serves to increase LBM; and, in the case of overnutrition, LBM

Table 1. Initial Values and Change with Exercise
means ± s.d. (range)

	N, sex	age	height (cm)	weight (kg)	LBM (kg)	arm circ. (cm)	av. skinfold (mm)
Group I							
Initial	11, M	(19–23)	180.4 ± 6.2 (169–190)	71.1 ± 6.2 (64–84)	61.5 ± 6.4 (51–73)	27.4 ± 1.5* (25.5–30.5)	7.7 ± 3.6* (5–16)
Change				−0.06 ± 1.1 (−2.3 to +1.2)	−0.61 ± 2.0 (−4.8 to +2.0)	+0.59 ± 0.69 (−0.5 to +1.5)	
Initial	4, F	(18–23)	165.8 (151–171)	58.8 (50–69)	45.6 (36–48)	25.2 ± 1.9 (22.6–27.0)	10.4** (8.6–18.3)
Change				−1.1 (−3.7 to +1.4)	−0− (−2.4 to +4.8)		−1.2 (−3.5 to +0.4)
Group II							
Initial	1, M	24	182	76.1	66.8	31.0	8.4
Change				+3.9	+3.4	−0−	+0.6
Initial	2, F	29, 19	160, 172	52.8, 70.0	39.1, 50.6	22.0, 27.8	11.4, 14.3
Change				0, +0.3	+3.1, +0.1	+1.0, +2.2	−0.7, —
Group III							
Initial	19, M	(19–21)	187.7 ± 4.6 (178–196)	94.9 ± 9.3 (74–106)	82.9 ± 5.7 (71–93)	35.3 ± 2.0 (32.5–39)	4.8 ± 0.9*** (3.5–6.6)
Change				−0.4 ± 2.2 (−6.2 to +2.7)	−0.8 ± 2.4 (−3.7 to +5.6)	−0.47 ± 0.72 (−1.0 to +1.5)	+0.3 ± 0.5 (−0.4 to +1.3)

*N = 8
**N = 3
***average biceps, triceps only

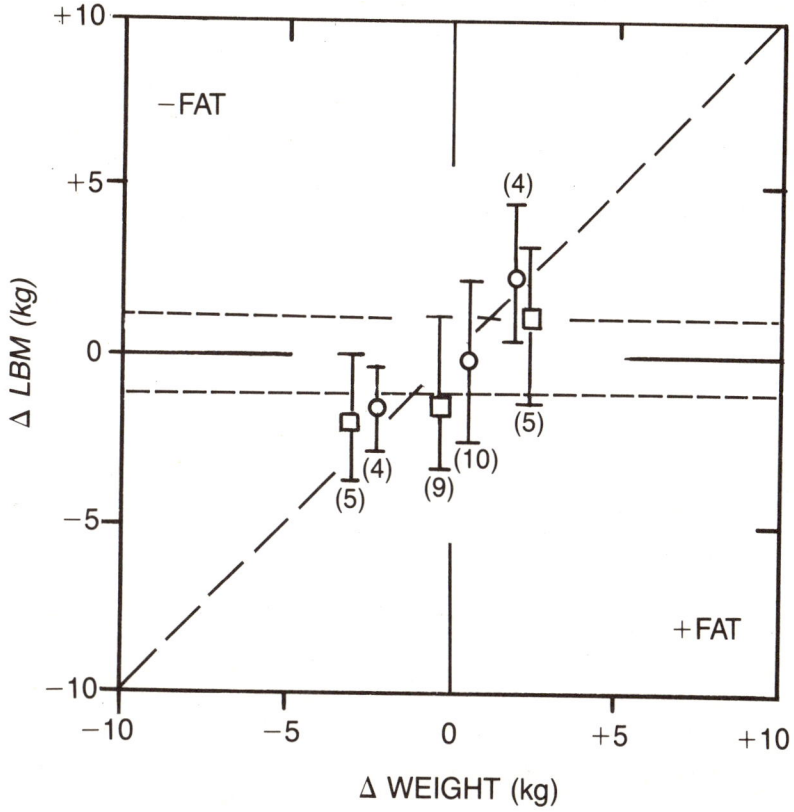

Figure 1. Plot of changes in LBM and weight subsequent to exercise in college students (○) and in football players (□). Subjects divided into three groups: those who lost one or more kg weight, those gaining at least one kg, and those whose weight changed less than one kg. Vertical bars show ± s.d.; horizontal dotted lines show replicability (s.d.) of LBM assay in absence of exercise or diet.

rises progressively with increasing obesity. While we have shown that obese males tend to have an increased LBM,[2] our data for them are not sufficient to permit the type of detailed analysis shown for females in Table 3.

The average weekly gain for the 50 pregnant women was 0.46 ± 0.13 (SD)kg and the average increment in LBM was 0.30 ± 0.13 kg. Hence, the calculated gain in body weight for the entire pregnancy was 13 kg, of which 8.4 kg represented LBM. These gains include the fetus and placenta which together weigh about 3.9 kg at term, and about 0.8 kg of amniotic fluid.[11] The total fat-free weight of these three components is about 4.3 kg and the total fat about 0.4 kg.[12] It is obvious that mother's body *per se* accumulates both LBM and fat during pregnancy.

Table 2. Group IV: Vigorous training, androgens

Subject	Age	Height (cm)	Weight (kg)	LBM (kg)	Fat (kg)	arm MB circ (cm)	av. Skinfold*** (mm)	Handgrip (kg)	
Weight lifter	31	176	107.4	80.6*	26.8	35.1	15.3	65	Pre-training
			112.9	96.6**	16.3	38.3	13.0	66	7 months training
			110.9	86.0**	24.9	37.0	16.4	68	Post-training 6 months
Body builder	27	179	94.9	86.9*	7.9	37.5	6.6	77	Pre-training
			107.1	103.4**	3.6	42.7	6.3	90	7 months training
			93.5	86.0**	7.3	39.6	6.6	77	Post-training 29 months

*average of 3 assays
**average of 2 assays
***biceps, triceps, subscapular, subcostal, umbilical, iliac

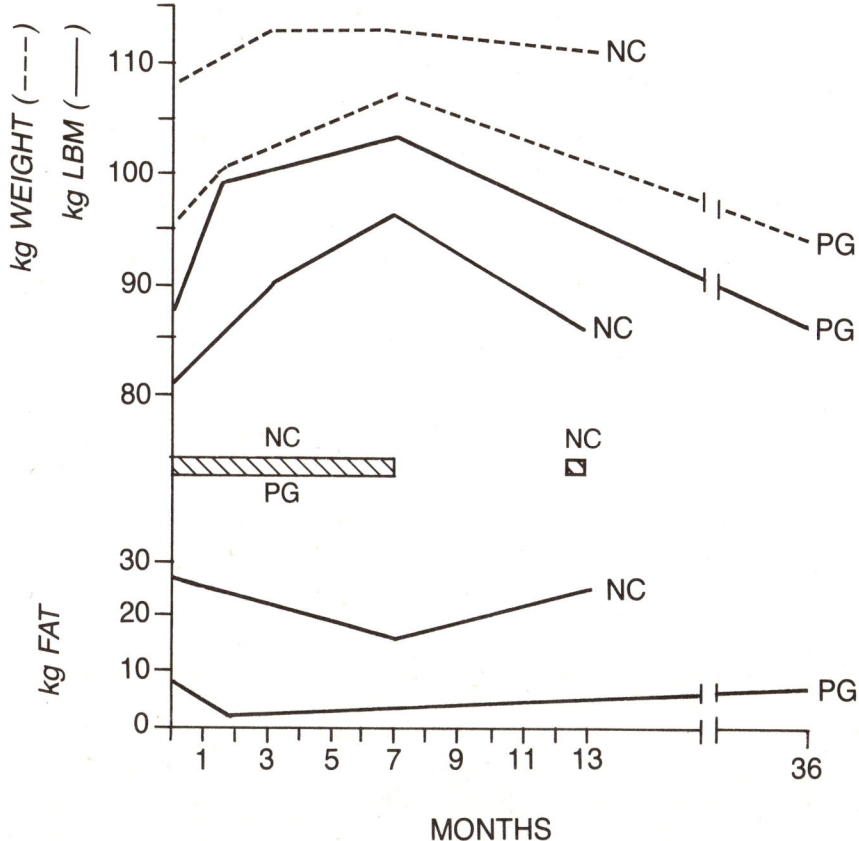

Figure 2. Changes in body weight, LBM, and body fat as a consequence of intense training and androgen administration. Upper section: body weight (- - -) and LBM (—); lower section: body fat. The bar indicates the period of training and medication.

Discussion

Exercise. Most of our exercising subjects (those presumably not taking androgens) did not experience an increase in LBM; indeed, only six of the 37 subjects had an increase of 2 kg or more. Figure 1 shows that the number of subjects who had a decrease in LBM approximated the number who had an increase. This disappointing result led to a critical review of the literature. Only those studies in which assays of body composition were done by ^{40}K counting, densitometry, or total body water are included. A variety of exercise and/or training programs are represented, including athletes assayed at the beginning of the competition season and either midway or at the end of the season.

Table 3. Female Subjects
(Author's data)

Subjects (N)	Body Fat (kg)	LBM (kg)
anorexia nervosa (10)	6.9 ± 2.6*	29.4 ± 4.7
normals (252)	13.8 ± 5.2	42.0 ± 4.8
normals (54)	19.4 ± 8.8	44.0 ± 5.5
mild obesity (12)	33.2 ± 3.8	51.3 ± 4.8
moderate obesity (6)	50.3 ± 4.2	57.2 ± 6.4
severe obesity (5)	75.9 ± 18	63.3 ± 4.8

*means ± s.d.

In Figure 3, the average changes in weight and LBM are plotted for the various exercising groups. An attempt was made to separate those athletes who engaged in moderate exercise for a few weeks from those who exercised more vigorously and/or for longer periods; the three groups of obese subjects are separately identified. Of the 24 groups portrayed, only four gained on average more than 2 kg LBM. For many of the groups, the recorded changes lie within the range of precision of the methods used to estimate LBM. One must conclude that exercise and/or training does not result in a significant augmentation in LBM for the majority of subjects thus far reported. Many years ago, Tanner[24] found that training did not lead to an increase in urinary creatinine excretion, and Parizkova[25] failed to observe an increase in LBM in rats who had exercised regularly for many weeks, though body fat was somewhat less than in controls.

It must be admitted, however, that the exercise programs employed by many investigators have not been very vigorous, nor of long duration. It would be of great interest to learn whether vigorous exercise on a long-term basis combined with adequate diet could significantly augment LBM in previously sedentary persons.

The fact that athletes tend to possess a larger LBM than sedentary individuals[3,25] is not proof that training *per se* accounts for the difference. Lean body mass does vary among normal individuals of the same age and sex[26]; hence, the athlete may have possessed a larger LBM from an early age, or possibly LBM could have been augmented through many years of training. The groups shown in Figure 3, with one exception, trained for only a few weeks or months. It is known that the winners of a number of Olympic events are taller than the average of all other participants in those events[27]; of significance here is the fact that LBM is in turn related to height.[1]

In considering what might be accomplished in altering body composition by exercise alone, one must keep in mind the limits inherent in the basic formula: Δ Wt = Δ LBM + Δ fat. The graph in Figure 4 shows the theoretical situation for two male subjects, each with 60 kg LBM, at the start of the exercise period; one with 25% body fat, the second with 15% body fat. If they set out to achieve a body fat content of 10%, ie, the fat content of a thin individual, the diagonal lines

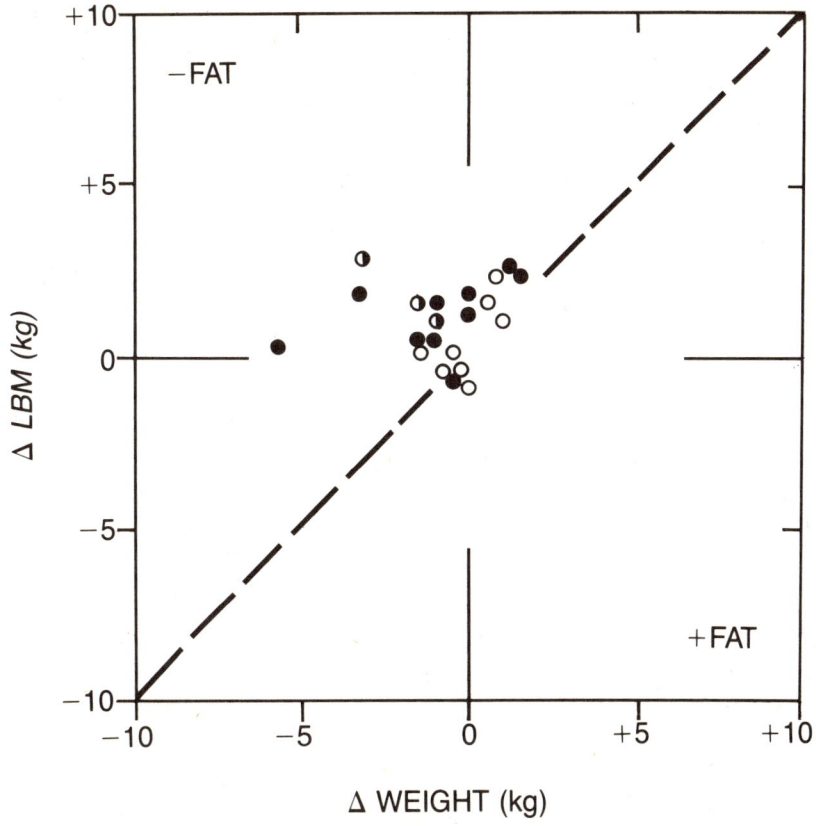

Figure 3. Effect of exercise and/or training on body weight and LBM. Group averages: ○—moderate exercise, data of Boileau et al,[13,14] Wilmore et al,[15,16] Hervey et al,[17] Ward,[18] Fahey and Brown,[19] Moody et al,[20] author's data (Table I). ●—vigorous training and/or exercise, data of Leon et al,[5] Carter and Phillips,[6] Kelly et al,[21] Parizkova,[4] Boddy et al,[22] Boileau et al,[14] Consolazio et al,[23] author's data (Table I). ◐—obese subjects, data of Boileau et al,[14] Moody et al.[20]

define the various combinations of changes in weight and LBM which can achieve that goal. If body weight does not change, these two subjects can gain no more than 12 and 3.5 kg LBM, respectively. Alternatively, if LBM is not to be lost, they can not lose more than 13.3 and 3.9 kg in weight, respectively. In the first situation, larger gains in LBM are possible only if body weight increases; in the second, larger losses in body weight will inevitably cause a decline in LBM. Any combination of changes in LBM and weight which are consistent with the stated goal of 10% body fat can be read off the diagonal lines.

Obviously, thin individuals who desire to substantially augment their lean weight by exercise should eat enough to increase body weight, since at a value of 10% body fat, LBM can not exceed 90% of body weight. The fatter the person, the more weight can be lost without adversely affecting LBM. In actuality, however, this statement may not hold true over an extended period of time since

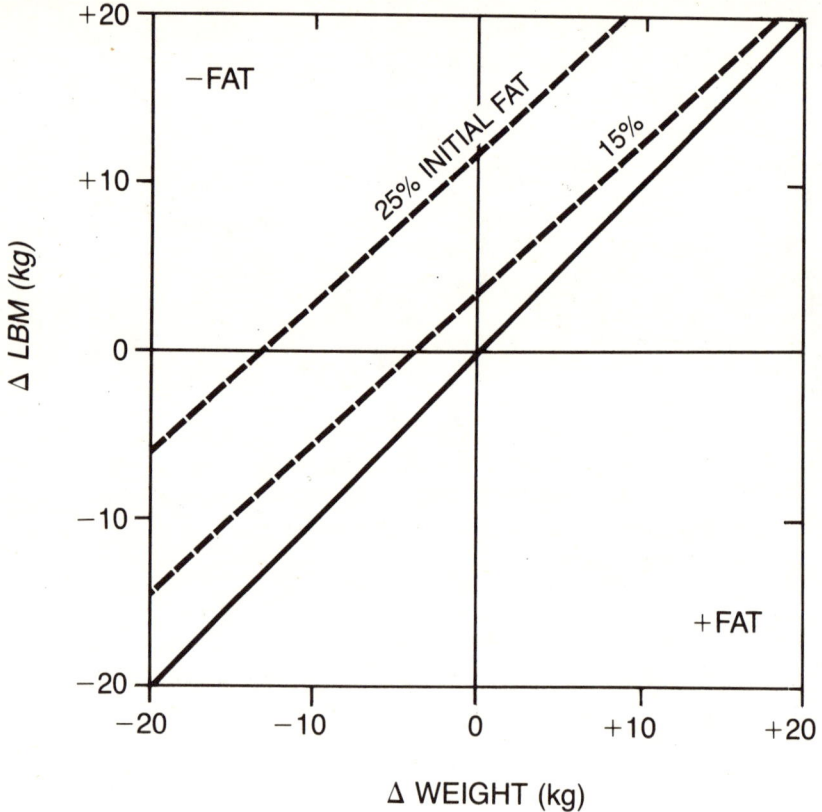

Figure 4. Plot of Δ against Δ weight, showing limits of change in LBM (dotted lines) for a given change in weight to achieve a final body fat content of 10%. Two theoretical male subjects are shown, one with initial body fat of 25% at the start of the exercise period, the other with 15% fat. The diagonal solid line shows Δ LBM for given Δ weight in the absence of a change in body fat. The region above this line indicates decrease in body fat and the region below indicates increase in fat.

the achievement of normal body composition through weight reduction by the obese would inevitably involve some loss of LBM (see Table 3). It remains to be seen whether vigorous and sustained exercise can forestall such an event.

Androgens. Rather striking effects are produced by changes in androgen levels. In males, androgen administration together with exercise leads to an increase in body weight and in LBM, and a decrease in body fat; the magnitude of the effect is roughly proportional to the dose of androgen and the duration of its administration (Table 4A, Figure 5). These results are not to be construed as advocating the use of androgens by athletes. Their use is known to interfere with gonadotropin production and with hepatic function, and to be accompanied by a fall in sperm count.[35]

The effects of subnormal (ie, for the male) androgen levels is seen both in the difference between normal and XXY males (the latter have serum testosterone

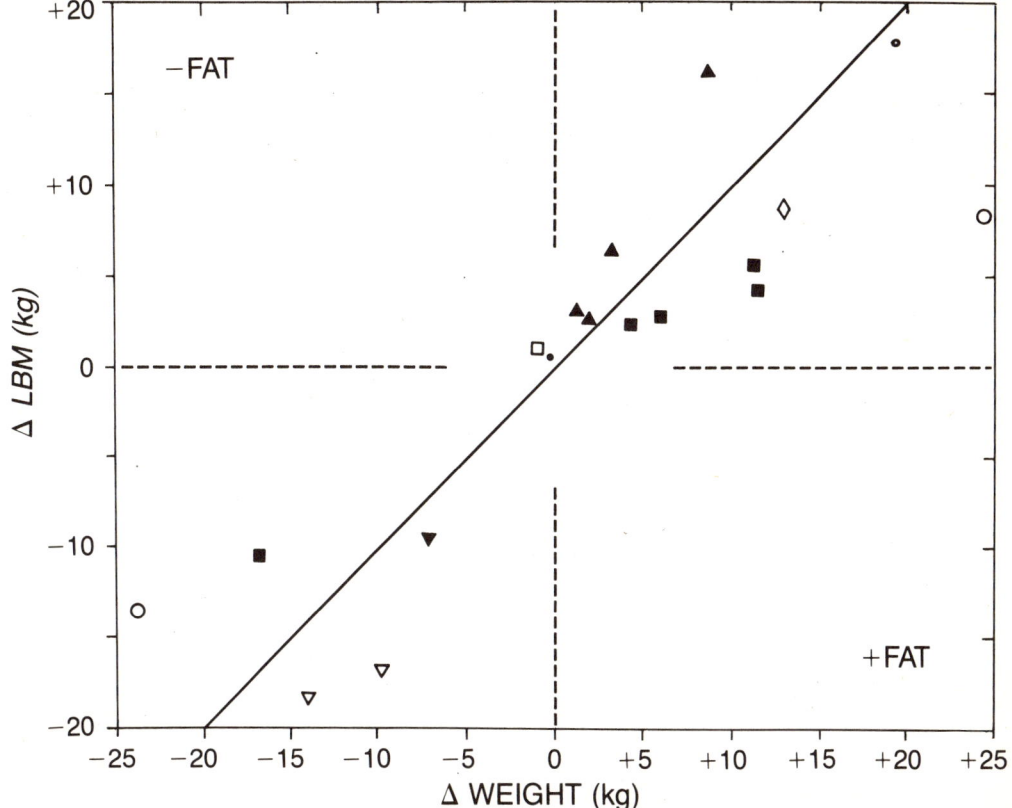

Figure 5. Plot of change in LBM against change in weight for various groups of subjects, showing effects of androgen levels, food intake, exercise, and pregnancy. Diagonal line shows LBM-weight relationship in absence of change in body fat; the region above this line indicates decrease in body fat, and below an increase in body fat. Influence of androgens: ▲—increments in LBM and weight resulting from androgen administration to males; ▼—difference between XXY and XY males; ▽—difference between late teenage females and males. Effects of nutrition: ■—results of deliberate underfeeding and overfeeding of males; ○—difference between anorexic and normal females, and between moderately obese and normal females. Effect of exercise (both sexes): ●—moderate exercise; □—vigorous exercise; ◇—changes during pregnancy. Data sources in Table 4A,B and legend for Figure 3.

levels midway between normal males and females[36]), and in the difference between normal young adult males and females. The same conclusion is reached if one chooses the young adult female as a starting point, ie, as androgen levels increase to those recorded for XXY males, to those in normal adults, and finally to males who take androgens, there is a progressive rise in body weight and in LBM, and a progressive fall in body fat.

The effect of androgens is also evident from the observation that the difference in body composition between adolescent males and females develops at about the same time that the sex difference in serum testosterone levels occur. By age

Table 4A. Data Sources for Figure 5 (averages)

Subjects	(N)	Procedure	Δ Weight (kg)	Δ LBM (kg)	Reference
Adult M	(8)	Androgens, exercise 5 wk	+ 1.3	+ 3.1	Ward[18]
Adult M	(7)	Androgens, exercise 6 wk	+ 2.3	+ 4.2	Hervey et al[28]
Adult M	(11)	Androgens, exercise 9 wk	+ 3.3	+ 6.3	Hervey et al[17]
Adult M	(14)	Androgens, exercise 9 wk	+ 2.1	+ 2.5	Fahey & Brown[19]
Adult M	(2)	Androgens, exercise 7 mo	+ 8.8	+ 16.2	Author's data
Adult M	(9)	Overfeeding 3 wk	+ 4.4	+ 2.5	Goldman et al[29]
Adult M	(6)	Overfeeding 6 wk	+ 6.0	+ 2.7	Norgan & Durnin[30]
Adult M	(4)	Overfeeding 12 wk	+ 11.2	+ 6.7	Goldman et al[29]
Adult M	(10)	Overfeeding 6 mo	+ 11.4	+ 4.2	Keys et al[31]
Adult M	(32)	Underfeeding, exercise	− 16.8	− 10.5	Keys & Brozek[32]
Adult M,F av. 9 groups		Moderate exercise	− 0.20	+ 0.47	See legend for Fig 3
Adult M,F av. 12 groups		Vigorous exercise	− 0.88	+ 1.06	See legend for Fig 3
Obese M,F av. 3 groups		Moderate exercise	− 1.8	+ 1.8	See legend for Fig 3

13 years, the male:female ratio for serum testosterone has risen from the childhood level of unity to approximately 2:1,[37] and it is at this age that the sex difference in LBM first becomes manifest.[26]

Nutrition. The effect of nutrition on LBM is also noteworthy. Not only do underweight persons (eg, patients with anorexia nervosa) have a reduced LBM, but Figure 5 also demonstrates that some LBM is lost through the deliberate underfeeding of individuals of normal weight. Both Ljunggren et al[38] and Davies et al[39] have reported that patients with anorexia nervosa have a reduced lean body weight as well as a lower body fat content. Conversely, both obesity (which can only develop via positive caloric balance) and deliberate overfeeding are associated with an increased LBM. The data in Table 3 show that LBM rises progressively with the degree of obesity (the values for the "moderate" and "severe" obese groups extend beyond the limits of Figure 5).

Hence, an increase in androgens (compared to normal levels in the adult male) leads to an increase in LBM and a decrease in fat, while reduced levels are associated with a smaller LBM and a larger amount of fat. Caloric excess, on the other hand, leads to an increase in *both* LBM and fat, whereas caloric deprivation leads to a decrease in both.

Figure 5 summarizes the available information from the literature and from the author's investigations. It depicts the effects of exercise and/or training, of food intake, and of androgens on body weight and LBM, and the changes which occur during normal pregnancy. Data sources for Figure 5 are given in Table 4A,B.

In summary, there appears to be an interplay of factors responsible for the status of body composition. The increase in weight and LBM recorded for the males who exercised and took androgens could not have been achieved without

Table 4B. Data Sources for Figure 5 (averages)

Subjects	(N)	Weight (kg)	LBM (kg)	Δ Weight (kg)	Δ LBM (kg)	Reference
Normal M	(23)	74.9	57.2			East et al[33]
XXY M	(10)	67.6	47.8	− 7.3	− 9.4	East et al[33]
Normal F	(306)	60.0	43.0			Author's data
Anorexic F	(10)	36.3	29.4	− 23.7	− 13.6	Author's data
Obese F	(12)	84.5	51.3	+ 24.5	+ 8.3	Author's data
Normal M*	(73)	70.5	61.1			Author's data
Normal F*	(68)	56.8	42.9	− 13.7	− 18.2	Author's data
Normal M**	(485)	67.6	56.9			Burmeister & Bingert[34]
Normal F**	(115)	57.8	40.1	− 9.8	− 16.8	Burmeister & Bingert[34]
Adult women (pregnant)	(50)			+ 13.0	+ 8.4	Author's data

* 17–20 years old
** 19–21 years old

an increase in caloric intake. On the other hand, the data in Figure 5 show that overfeeding alone could not have been responsible for the marked rise in LBM; nor for that matter, could exercise alone have brought it about. Several investigators[17-19] have found that the LBM of subjects on identical exercise programs did not increase to the extent seen with androgen administration. The basic reason(s) for the increase in LBM recorded for the overfed males and the obese females is not known. The increased plasma insulin levels and the increased urinary excretion of 17-ketosteroids, both of which occur in spontaneous as well as in induced obesity,[40] suggest that hormone action could facilitate this process.

Pregnancy. This situation represents such an interplay of factors since the increased food intake is superimposed on an elevation in the serum levels of a number of hormones: insulin, placental lactogen, progesterone, prolactin, testosterone, androstenedione, and estrogens.[41,42] Some of these are androgenic, and some have growth hormone-like actions. This may account for the fact that the proportion of weight gain due to LBM is relatively greater in pregnancy than that recorded for simple overnutrition. This was demonstrated by our findings and those of Seitchik.[43]

Summary

Sufficient data are now available with which to discern the effects of exercise, androgens, pregnancy, and nutrition on body composition in man. Androgen excess increases lean body mass (LBM) and weight, and decreases body fat; when compared to normal androgen levels in males, lower androgen levels are associated with a smaller LBM and a larger body fat content. Energy excess increases LBM, weight, and fat; energy deficiency reverses the process. Although some body fat can be lost through exercise, the effect on LBM is very modest.

Pregnancy leads to an increase in both LBM and fat, but proportionately more of the LBM than does simple overnutrition.

Acknowledgments

Supported by NIH grants HD-18454 and RR00044, and based on work performed under Contract No. DE-AC02-76-EVO-3490 with the US Department of Energy at the University of Rochester Department of Radiation Biology and Biophysics and has been assigned Report No. UR-3490-2019.

The assistance of Eulalia Halloran, Cheryl Porta, and Kathleen Morris is gratefully acknowledged.

References

1. Forbes GB: Stature and lean body mass. *Am J Clin Nutr* 27:1073–1079, 1974.
2. Forbes GB: Lean body mass and fat in obese children. *Pediatrics* 34:308–314, 1964.
3. Behnke AR, Wilmore JH: *Evaluation and Regulation of Body Build and Composition*, Englewood Cliffs, NJ, Prentice-Hall, Inc, 1974.
4. Parizkova J: Impact of age, diet, and exercise on man's body composition. *Ann NY Acad Sci*:110, 661–674, 1963.
5. Leon AS, Conrad J, Hunninghake DB, et al: Effects of a vigorous walking program on body composition, and lipid metabolism of obese young men. *Am J Clin Nutr* 32:1776–1787, 1979.
6. Carter JEL, Phillips WH: Structural changes in exercising middle-aged males during a 2-year period. *J Appl Physiol* 27:787–794, 1969.
7. Nelson EA, Craig AB, Jr: Physiologic responses to a transcontinental bicycle trip. *Physicians and Sports Med* 6: No. 6, June 1978.
8. Forbes GB, Schultz F, Cafarelli C, et al: Effects of body size on potassium-40 measurements in the whole body counter (tilt-chair technique). *Health Phys* 15:435–442, 1968.
9. Forbes GB: Methods for determining composition of the human body. *Pediatrics* 29:477–494, 1962.
10. Landau RL: The metabolic effects of anabolic steroids in man, in Kochakian CD (ed): *Anabolic-androgenic Steroids*, New York, Springer-Verlag, 1976, pp 45–72.
11. Hytten FE, Leitch I: *The Physiology of Human Pregnancy*, 2nd ed, Oxford, England, Blackwell, 1971, p 269.
12. Widdowson EM, Spray CM: Chemical development *in utero*. *Arch Dis Child* 26:205–214, 1951.
13. Boileau RA, Massey BH, Misner JE: Body composition changes in adult men during selected weight training and jogging programs. *Res Q* 44:158–168, 1963.
14. Boileau RA, Buskirk ER, Horstman DH, et al: Body composition changes in obese and lean men during physical conditioning. *Med Sci Sports* 3:183–189, 1971.
15. Wilmore JH, Girandola R, Katch F, et al: Body composition changes with a 10-week program of jogging. *Med Sci Sports* 2:113–117, 1970.
16. Wilmore JH, Davis JA, O'Brien RS, et al: Physiological alterations consequent to 20 week conditioning programs of bicycling, tennis and jogging. *Med Sci Sports* 12:1–8, 1980.
17. Hervey GR, Hutchinson I, Knibbs AV, et al: "Anabolic" effects of methandienone in men undergoing athletic training. *Lancet* 2:699–702, 1976.
18. Ward P: The effect of an anabolic steroid on strength and lean body mass. *Med Sci Sports* 5:277–282, 1973.
19. Fahey TD, Brown CH: The effects of an anabolic steroid on the strength, body composition, and endurance of college males when accompanied by a weight training program. *Med Sci Sports* 5:272–276, 1973.
20. Moody DL, Wilmore JH, Girandola RN, et al: The effects of a jogging program on the body composition of normal and obese high school girls. *Med Sci Sports* 4:210, 1972.
21. Kelly JM, Gorney BA, Kalm KK: The effects of a collegiate wrestling season on body composition, cardiovascular fitness and muscular strength and endurance. *Med Sci Sports* 10:119–124, 1978.

22. Boddy K, Hume R, King PC, et al: Total body, plasma and erythrocyte potassium and leucocyte ascorbic acid in 'ultra-fit' subjects. *Clin Sci Mol Med* 46:449–456, 1974.

23. Consolazio CF, Johnson HL, Nelson RA, et al: Protein metabolism during intensive physical training in the young adult. *Am J Clin Nutr* 28:29–35, 1975.

24. Tanner JM: The effect of weight-training on physique. *Am J Phys Anthropol* 10:427–461, 1952.

25. Parizkova, J: *Body Fat and Physical Fitness*. The Hague, M. Nijhoff, B.V., 1977, p. 68.

26. Forbes GB: Growth of the lean body mass in man. *Growth* 36:325–338, 1972.

27. Khosla T: Unfairness of certain events in the Olympic Games. *Br Med J* 4:111–113, 1968.

28. Hervey GR, Knibbs AV, Burkinshaw L, et al: Effects of methandienone on the performance and body composition of men undergoing athletic training. *Clin Sci Mol Med* 60:457–461, 1981.

29. Goldman RF, Haisman MF, Bynum G, et al: Experimental obesity in man: metabolic rate in relation to dietary intake, in Bray GA (ed): *Obesity in Perspective*, US Department of Health, Education and Welfare Publication No (NIH) 75–708, 1975, pp 165–186.

30. Norgan NG, Durnin JV: The effect of 6 weeks of overfeeding on the body weight, body composition, and energy metabolism of young men. *Am J Clin Nutr* 33:978–988, 1980.

31. Keys A, Anderson JT, Brozek J: Weight gain from simple overeating. *Metabolism* 4:427–432, 1955.

32. Keys A, Brozek J: Body fat in adult man. *Physiol Rev* 33:245–325, 1953.

33. East BW, Boddy K, Price WH: Total body potassium content in males with X and Y chromosome abnormalities. *Clin Endocrinol* 5:43–51, 1976.

34. Burmeister W, Bingert A: Die quantitativen Veränderungen der menschlichen Zellmasse zwischen dem 8 und 90 Lebensjahr. *Klin Wochenschr* 45:409–416, 1967.

35. Weintraub M, Horvitz R: The effects of high dose anabolic steroids on the response to clomiphene and LHRF. *Pharmacologist* 16:319, 1974.

36. Paulsen CA, Gordon DL, Carpenter RW: Klinefelter's syndrome and its variants: a hormonal and chromosomal study. *Recent Prog Horm Res* 24:321–363, 1968.

37. Winter JSD: Prepubertal and pubertal endocrinology, in Falkner F, Tanner JM (eds): *Human Growth*, vol. 2, New York, Plenum Press, 1978, pp 183–213.

38. Ljunggren H, Ikkos D, Luft R: Studies on body composition. *Acta Endocrinol* 25:209–223, 1957.

39. Davies CTM, von Döbeln W, Fohlin L, et al: Total body potassium, fat free weight and maximal aerobic power in children with anorexia nervosa. *Acta Paediatr Scand* 67:229–234, 1978.

40. Bray GA, *The Obese Patient*. Philadelphia, W.B. Saunders Co. 1976, pp 252–299.

41. Buster JE, Marshall JR: Conception, gamete and ovum transport, implantation, fetal-placental hormones, hormonal preparation for parturition and parturition control, in De Groot LJ, et al (eds): *Endocrinology*, vol. 3, New York, Grune & Stratton, 1979, pp. 1595–1612.

42. Levitz M: Steroid metabolism in the fetal-placental-maternal unit, in Iffy L, Kaminetsky HA: (eds): *Principles and Practice of Obstetrics*, New York, John Wiley & Sons, 1981, pp. 261–267.

43. Seitchik J.: Total body water and total body density of pregnant women. *Obstet Gyn* 29:155–166, 1967.

INTERRELATION OF PHYSICAL ACTIVITY AND NUTRITION ON OBESITY

Per Björntorp, MD*

The subject of this paper encompasses a vast area, and in order to focus this brief review on what appears to be the core of the matter, the following aspects of the problem have been selected for discussion. First, the question of weight decrease during exercise programs will be examined. What is the explanation for the decrease in weight? Second, the potential for additional benefit from exercise when combined with a diet program will be considered. Diet alone as treatment of obesity will essentially be omitted from this review, being an impossible area to cover in a limited space. The review will not cover totally the published works in the areas discussed. The references have been mainly selected to illustrate the opinion of the author based on other publications not referred to in this paper.

Effect of Exercise on Body Weight

Exercise does cause a decrease of body weight without alterations in the diet. The fact that athletes engaged in endurance sports are thin is well established. Longitudinal observations show that skinfolds decrease during training periods without any restriction in dietary intake.[1] A similar phenomenon has been observed also in less extreme situations and in a less selected population who are not obese or are slightly obese.[2] There are also numerous reports showing that a weight decrease is obtained in obese patients. Oscai and Williams[3] found a decrease of about 4 kg body fat in men who jogged 30 minutes per day, three times per week, for approximately four months. Gwinup[4] succeeded in obtaining a weight reduction in obese subjects who had previously failed to maintain weight loss after dieting.

There is, however, an interesting exception to this general rule in severely obese subjects with hyperplastic adipose tissue; body fat in these individuals decreases very slowly or not at all with exercise.[5,6] Possible explanations to this phenomenon will be discussed in another section of this paper.

The question then arises: Why does body fat decrease during a continuous exercise program? In principle, this could be due either to increased energy expenditure or to decreased energy intake or both.

Obviously, there is an increase of energy output during an exercise program; however, the extra expended energy during the exercise sessions is surprisingly small, amounting usually to a few hundred calories. In studies where the expended energy during the exercise sessions can be quantitated with reason-

---

*Sahlgren's Hospital, University of Goteborg, Sweden

able certainty and compared with the loss of body fat, it can be calculated that this extra energy output can not cover the entire loss of body energy.[2,7] The report of Oscai and Williams[3] lends further support to such a conclusion. The men jogged for about 30 minutes, three times per week, which amounts to an energy expenditure of approximately 1000 kcal. During the period of the study (16 weeks), they should have lost about 16,000 kcal or little more than 2 kg body fat; however, they lost about 4 kg. Provided energy intake did not change, observations of this type suggest additional mechanisms may account for body fat loss during exercise programs.

The most obvious and most studied explanation for a decrease of body fat during exercise programs is the effect of exercise on energy intake. The most frequently cited work is that of Mayer et al[8] who compared sedentary rats with exercising rats and found that the sedentary rats ate more than the exercising animals. At a certain point in the duration of the exercise, however, the exercising rats compensated for the expended energy by extra food intake, keeping the body weight constant at a lower level than in the sedentary condition. This work has, in essence, been confirmed by other studies. There are, however, variations in this uniform picture caused by the intensity and duration of exercise. Exercise of high intensity and short duration is more effective in decreasing body fat than is low intensity exercise of long duration. Furthermore, there seems to be a sex difference, male rats responding more effectively than female rats.[9]

Although results in studies in the rat seem reasonably conclusive, the information in man is much less clear. The initial study of Mayer et al[10] in an industrial male population was suggested to show analogous results as the corresponding study in the rat, but this conclusion can be criticized.[11] A number of other studies show varying results. In most of these studies, it is difficult to evaluate the energy balance in terms of exactly controlled energy output and the resulting changes in body composition. In addition, the precision of measuring energy intake that is voluntarily changed is by necessity limited.

A recent study has examined this important question during strictly controlled conditions as far as is practically possible.[12] The food intake, measured in a metabolic ward, was carefully monitored and the energy expenditure was measured during a long-term exercise program of low and high intensity. Changes in body composition were followed by several techniques. There was no evidence that exercise caused an inhibition of energy intake.

As seen from this brief summary, the data from human studies do not show an inhibitory effect of exercise on energy intake; however, the information is not yet conclusive.

The remaining factor in the energy balance equation is the effect of exercise on thermogenetic factors. There is some direct and indirect evidence available on this point. Measurements of thyroid hormones in circulation seem to provide little information. Although the literature is inconsistent, it appears that exercise training seems to have a similar effect on hormone concentrations as does energy intake restrictions.[13]

Energy expenditure is elevated not only during exercise but also for a period of time after. This period probably varies depending on the degree of physical conditioning; for example, the circulatory steady state is reached earlier in well-trained subjects than in sedentary subjects and the "oxygen debt" is smaller. Reports of the duration of such increased oxygen uptake indicate that this effect of exercise continues after the circulatory steady state has been reached. For example, Edwards et al[14] reported a 10 percent elevation of basal metabolic rate for as long as 48 hours after exercise. Clearly, such phenomena would add to the energy cost of exercise and contribute to body fat loss more than the energy expended during the exercise period alone.

The question of a more constant activation of thermogenetic processes by exercise training does not seem to have been tested directly. The fact that the adrenergic nervous system is involved in the activation of these processes makes it of particular interest to examine the effects physical training might have on this activity. In the steady state, the excretion of epinephrine and norepinephrine does not change with physical training in both obese and nonobese subjects.[6] On the other hand, there is evidence of an increased sensitivity in different parts of the adrenergic nervous system, including circulation, insulin secretion and lipolytic response.[15-17] Whether a similar effect is achieved in the area of the adrenergic nervous system that regulates the thermogenetic energy output is a question of high priority for future research and is at present an attractive hypothesis.

As noted earlier, exercise in obese individuals is usually followed by a diminution of body fat stores. There are, however, exceptions as found in subjects characterized by a severe hyperplastic obesity.[5,6] This finding might be indicative of a basic error in the energy balance of such obese subjects. If we look at the three forenamed possibilities to explain the body fat decrease that usually occurs in moderately obese or nonobese subjects, then differences in actual expenditure of energy during exercise is not a factor to consider because extremely heavy subjects expend more energy on a given exercise than nonobese or moderately obese subjects. The effects of exercise on energy intake are uncertain. One potential explanation for the unexpected lack of decrease in body fat, or even an occasional increase,[5] in such patients during exercise is the factor of overeating. Another alternative is a deficient adaptation of a thermogenetic adaptation to exercise. Clearly, this is an area for further research that would be of great interest.

Regional Effects of Physical Training on Adipose Tissue

A question of great public interest is: How does physical training affect the different regions of adipose tissue? Anecdotal evidence has indicated that fat tissue above a working muscle would decrease preferentially. This question has recently been tested with a one-leg exercise study, the inactive leg being used as a control. The results showed a somewhat thinner subcutaneous adipose tissue over the trained femoral muscle groups. Since the fat cells contained the same amount of triglyceride,[18] the result was due to a stretching of this tissue over a larger cylinder of muscle after training and not to an emptying of the depot. The end result might be considered as cosmetically desirable, but there was no evidence of a decrease in the local triglyceride store.

Clearly, different regions of adipose tissue are subject to the influence of hormones in a specific way. There is conclusive evidence for this statement in studies in the rat.[19] In humans, it seems reasonably clear that female sex hormones tend to "protect" the triglyceride content of the adipocytes in the gluteal-femoral regions. Young women specifically have larger fat cells in this region than do young men,[20] although estrogen treatment of men produces specific accumulation of adipocyte triglycerides here.[21] This corresponds to findings of less metabolically active adipocytes in these regions; for example, the lipolytic response is blunted.[22] Abdominal fat cells, on the other hand, seem more sensitive to energy balance changes, and are more responsive to the main hormones for lipid accumulation and release.[22,23] Although not studied as yet, the consequences of these characteristic regional adipocyte functions might well be that the decrease of the adipose depot caused by physical training is more pronounced in certain regions than in others. Given the information available, it appears that the adipocytes in the abdominal region would decrease more rapidly than the adipocytes in the gluteal-femoral regions in women. The latter regions are of considerable relative magnitude in most women, which may result in women having more difficulties than men in decreasing total body fat during physical training. This is reminiscent of the findings of differences in weight decreases among male and female rats mentioned earlier. Clearly, this is a question of large practical and public interest which needs more direct studies.

Effect of Exercise and Diet on Body Fat of Obese Individuals

The two main questions of interest here are whether or not exercise produces additional weight decrease during a diet program, and whether the loss of nitrogen and lean body mass occurring with low-calorie diets can be prevented with exercise.

Buskirk et al[24] found that exercise plus diet was more effective on weight loss than diet alone. There are a number of reports with similar conclusions.[25,26] The first question can, in all likelihood, be answered affirmatively. In this regard, however, it must be mentioned that strict, long-term, low-energy diets might make it difficult to maintain a strenuous exercise program, particularly for severely obese subjects who might be restricted in activity by the condition itself. Close guidance, observation, and encouragement, as well as individualized programs, might be needed.

In a combined program of diet and exercise, it is important to measure not only the decrease in gross body weight but to include measurements of body cell mass and body fat separately. An increase in body cell mass caused by the exercise would tend to mask a decrease in body fat, particularly since muscle has a higher density than fat. In most studies where exercise and diet have been used as combined treatment for obesity, these body compartments have not been measured separately; therefore, a saving effect of exercise on body cell mass can not be evaluated here. There are, however, exceptions. One study suggests that exercise spares the protein stores which a low-calorie diet tends to diminish.[26] Other studies,[28] however, do not give indications of decreased nitrogen loss during treatment which combines diet and exercise as compared to diet alone. This question must, at present, be considered unresolved.

It is clear that an organism on a continuous low-energy diet spares energy by diminution of oxygen consumption and thermogenesis. This probably occurs to a varying extent in different obese subjects under treatment, and seems to virtually prevent successful weight reduction after a period of time in some patients. Clearly, counteracting such sparing of energy would be highly desirable in the treatment of obesity. The question is: What effect does exercise have here?

Some studies have addressed this question, unfortunately with different results. Stern et al[29] reported that the decrease in basal metabolic rate (BMR) and triodothyronine (T3) caused by a low caloric diet was halted and tended to return to baseline when exercise was added to the program. Toss et al[30] were unable to find such an effect of exercise. The reasons for the discrepancies are not clear. The specific time when measurements are made in relation to the exercise sessions might, for example, be one factor. Future research on this important question is needed and will hopefully resolve these problems. The question is of particular interest because in analogy with weight decrease achieved by exercise *alone*, the weight loss achieved by exercise *with* dieting might well be greater than that expected from the extra energy expenditure during the exercise sessions.

Summary

Exercise without dieting causes a decrease in body fat, except in severely hyperplastic obese subjects. It seems that such decrease in body fat can not be explained fully by the increase in energy expenditure during the exercise sessions, an amount of energy which is usually limited. Contributory factors here are probably a protracted increase in energy expenditure *after* cessation of the exercise sessions. It is also possible that a sensitization of thermogenetic responses occurs through catecholamine mediation; there is evidence for an increased catecholamine sensitivity after physical training.

Another reason for loss of body fat during exercise programs is the effect of such exercise on energy intake. Although it seems clear that exercise inhibits energy intake in the rat, the evidence in man does not allow a similar conclusion at present.

The decrease in body fat in severely obese subjects engaged in exercise programs is abnormally slow. This fact might hide a basic regulatory error either in the regulation of appetite or, perhaps more likely, in energy output regulation.

Of practical importance is the question of regional loss of body fat with exercise. Although direct evidence is lacking, it appears that exercise is less effective in decreasing the adipose depot in regions protected by specific sex hormonal effect, eg, the gluteal-femoral region in women, than in other regions of the body. Sex differences in response to physical training are insufficiently understood.

There is conclusive evidence that exercise added to dietary programs for treatment of obesity has an additional effect on decrease of body weight. It is uncertain whether body cell mass can be spared. Whether or not the decreased thermogenesis that occurs during energy deficiency can be reversed by exercise is not yet clear.

References

1. Parizkova J, Poupa O: Some metabolic consequences of adaptation to muscular work. *Brit J Nutr* 17:341–345, 1963.
2. Bjorntorp P, Berchtold P, Grimby G, et al: Effects of physical training on glucose tolerance, plasma, insulin, and lipids, and on body composition in men after myocardial infarction. *Acta Med Scand* 192:439–443, 1972.
3. Oscai LB, Williams BT: Effect of exercise on overweight middle-aged males. *J Am Geriatr Soc* 16:794–797, 1968.
4. Gwinup G: Effects of exercise alone on the weight of obese women. *Arch Intern Med* 135:676–680, 1975.
5. Bjorntorp P, de Jounge K, Sjostrom L, et al: The effect of physical training on insulin production in obesity. *Metabolism* 19:631–636, 1970.
6. Bjorntorp P, de Jounge K, Krotkiewski M, et al: Physical training in human obesity III. Effects of long-term physical training on body composition. *Metabolism* 22:1467–1472, 1973.
7. Bjorntorp P: Exercise in the treatment of obesity. *Clin Endocrin Metab* 5:(2)431–453, 1976.
8. Mayer J, Marshall NB, Vitale JJ, et al: Exercise, food intake, and body weight in normal rats and genetically obese adult mice. *Am J Physiol* 177:544–548, 1954.
9. Oscai LB, Molé PA, Krusack LM, et al: Detailed body composition analysis on female rats subjected to a program of swimming. *J Nutr* 103:412–418, 1973.
10. Mayer J, Roy P, Mitra KP: Relation between caloric intake, body weight, and physical work: Studies in an industrial male population in West Bengal. *Am J Clin Nutr* 4:169–175, 1956.
11. Garrow, JS: *Energy Balance and Obesity in Man*. New York: Elsevier North-Holland, Inc., 1978a.
12. Pi-Sunyer X, Wu R, Garrow RS: (personal communication, 1981).
13. Wirth A, Holm G, Lindstedt G, et al: Thyroid hormones and lipolysis in physically trained rats. *Metabolism* 30:237–241, 1981.
14. Edwards HT, Thorndike A, Dill DB: The energy requirement in strenuous exercise. *N Engl J Med* 213:532–535, 1935.
15. Krotkiewski M, William-Olsson T, Bjorntorp P: Increased B-adrenergic sensitivity after physical training. In preparation.
16. Askey EW, Huston RL, Popper CG, et al: Adipose tissue cellularity and lipolysis. Response to exercise and cortisol treatment. *J Clin Invest* 56:521–529, 1975.
17. Holm G, Jacobsson B, Toss L, et al: The effect of physical exercise on the regulation of beta adrenergic receptors and adenylate cyclase in rat adipocytes. *Alimentazione, Nutrizione, Metabolismo* 1:280, 1980.
18. Krotkiewski M, Aniansson A, Grimby G, et al: The effect of unilateral isokinetic strength training on local adipose and muscle tissue morphology, thickness and enzymes. *Eur J Appl Physiol* 22:221–279, 1979.
19. Krotkiewski M, Bjorntorp P: The effect of progesterone and of insulin administration in regional adipose tissue cellularity in the rat. *Acta Physiol Scand* 96:122–126, 1976.
20. Sjostrom L, Smith U, Krotkiewski M, et al: Cellularity in different regions of adipose tissue in young men and women. *Metabolism* 21:1143–47, 1972.

21. Krotkiewski M, Bjorntorp P: The effects of estrogen treatment of carcinoma of the prostrate on regional adipocyte size. *J Endocrinol Invest* 365–368, 1978.

22. Smith U, Hammarsten J, Bjorntorp P, et al: Regional differences and effect of weight reduction on human fat cell metabolism. *Eur J Clin Invest* 9:323–333, 1979.

23. Krotkiewski M, Sjostrom L, Bjorntorp P, et al: Regional adipose tissue cellularity in relation to metabolism in young and middle-aged women. *Metabolism* 24:703–707, 1975.

24. Buskirk ER, Thompson RH, Lutwak L, et al: Energy balance in obese patients during weight reduction: influence of diet restriction and exercise. *Ann NY Acad Sci* 110:918–940, 1963.

25. Kenrick MM, Ball MF, Canary JJ: Exercise and weight reduction in obesity. *Arch Phys Med Rehabil* 53:323–327, 1972.

26. Zuti WB, Golding LA: Comparing diet and exercise as weight reduction tools. *Physician and Sports Medicine* 4:49–53, 1976.

27. Foss ML, Lampman RM, Schteingart DE: Extremely obese patients: improvements in exercise tolerance with physical training and weight loss. *Arch Phys Med Rehabil* 61:119–124, 1980.

28. Warwick PM, Garrow JS: The effect of addition of exercise to a regime of dietary restriction on weight loss, nitrogen balance, resting metabolic rate and spontaneous physical activity in three obese women in a metabolic ward. *Internat J Obesity* 5:25, 1981.

29. Stern JS, Schultz C, Mole P, et al: Effect of caloric restriction and exercise on basal metabolism and thyroid hormone. *Alimentazione, Nutrizione, Metabolismo* 1:361, 1980.

30. Toss L, Krotkiewski M, Lindstedt G, et al: Thyroid hormones and sex hormone binding globulin (SHBG) in obese patients treated with low energy intake with or without exercise. *Alimentazione, Nutrizione, Metabolismo* 1:369, 1980.

INTERRELATION OF PHYSICAL ACTIVITY AND NUTRITION ON BONE MASS

G. Donald Whedon, MD*

Introduction

Review of the literature over recent years shows that very few studies have been done which reflect specifically on the interrelated effects of physical activity *and* manipulations of dietary intake on bone mass. Thus, deductions must be drawn mainly from data on the effects of positive and negative physical activity *per se* on bone and from data on the effects of nutrition *per se* on bone, principally from changes in the intake level of calcium. Specific studies of the interrelation of diet and physical activity on bone mass are limited to attempts to determine whether increasing the calcium intake would have a diminishing effect on the degree of bone mass loss brought about by inactivity.

In this review, it is necessary to define the measurement of bone mass. Changes in bone mass will be ascribed to changes in total bone calcium (TB Ca) as measured by neutron activation, to changes in regional amounts of bone as measured by photon absorptiometry (BMC) of the radius or os calcis, or to regional changes by radiogrammetry (cortical thickness in relation to width of the whole bone as measured on a roentgenogram). If we are to have sufficient studies to draw some conclusions, however, we must also include changes in calcium balance, if large enough and measured long enough, as indicative of changes in bone mass. Changes in calcium balance surveyed in this report may have been measured by careful control of intake and collection of output or calculated from isotopic kinetic studies. Techniques of actual measurement of bone mass, or bone mineral content, are still in development and have been used only in recent research. In defining terms, it must also be borne in mind that regional mass measurements in the radius, which read predominantly cortical bone, correlate only variably with observations of the axial skeleton or with whole body mineral.

Effects of Physical Inactivity

More detailed data are available on the effects of inactivity on bone than are available on the effects of increased activity. Prior to the development of true mass measurement techniques, the technique of careful, continuous metabolic balance was used to discover and define the hypercalciuria and total loss of

---

*National Institute of Arthritis, Diabetes, and Digestive and Kidney Diseases, National Institutes of Health, Bethesda, Maryland

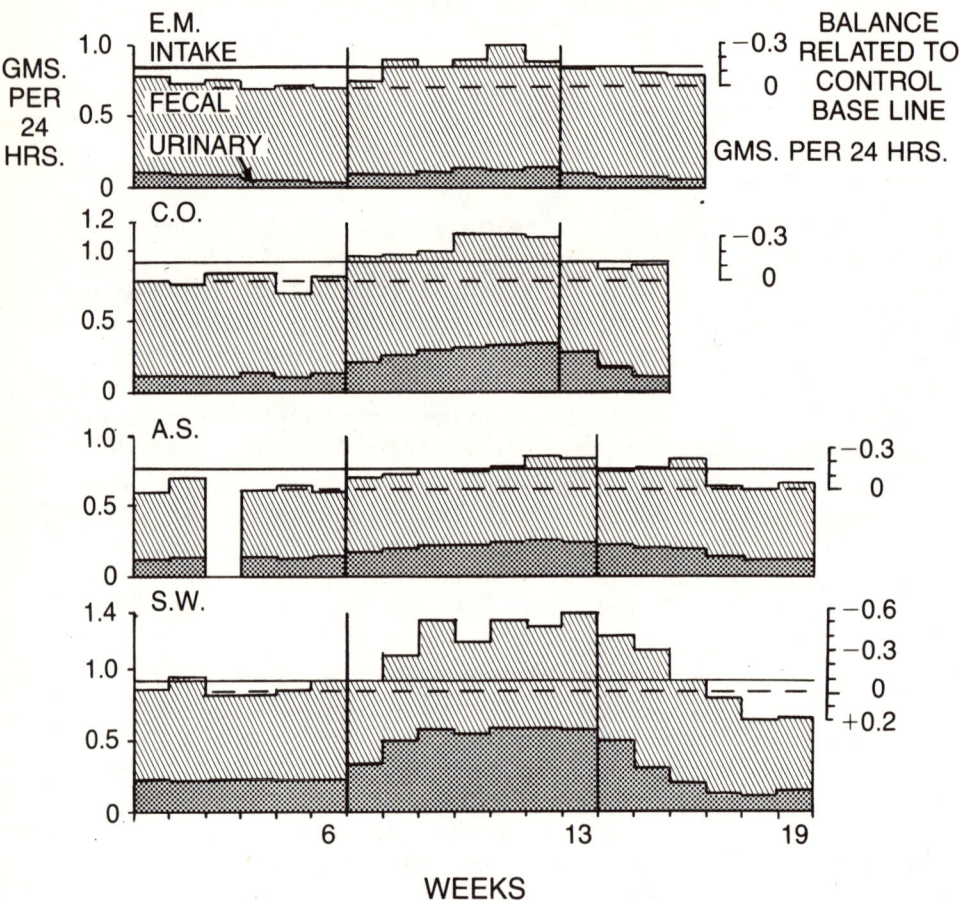

Figure 1. Effect of immobilization on calcium metabolism of four normal male subjects. In each subject the daily calcium intake was kept constant throughout all periods of the experiment. For each subject the control base-line (interrupted horizontal line) is an average of the total outputs of the last four control weeks.[1]

calcium from the body of normal human subjects who were immobilized (Figure 1).[1] The loss of mineral continued for the duration of immobilization and then gradually subsided upon resumption of ambulation. In paralytic poliomyelitis,[2] a similar pattern was observed but to a greater degree. Loss of calcium continued to the point of bone loss that was visible by ordinary roentgenogram.

More recently, extended studies of normal subjects at bed rest have been conducted (Figure 2).[3] Calcium loss did not subside until the subjects were ambulatory. In these latter studies, loss of bone mass was demonstrated by photon absorptiometry scans of the os calcis; on re-ambulation, the density of the heel bone was restored to normal.

Similar losses of calcium from the skeleton were observed in metabolic studies of the astronauts in the Skylab space flights (Figure 3)[4]; significant decreases in os calcis density were observed in the three astronauts who lost the greatest amounts of calcium in the balance studies.[5]

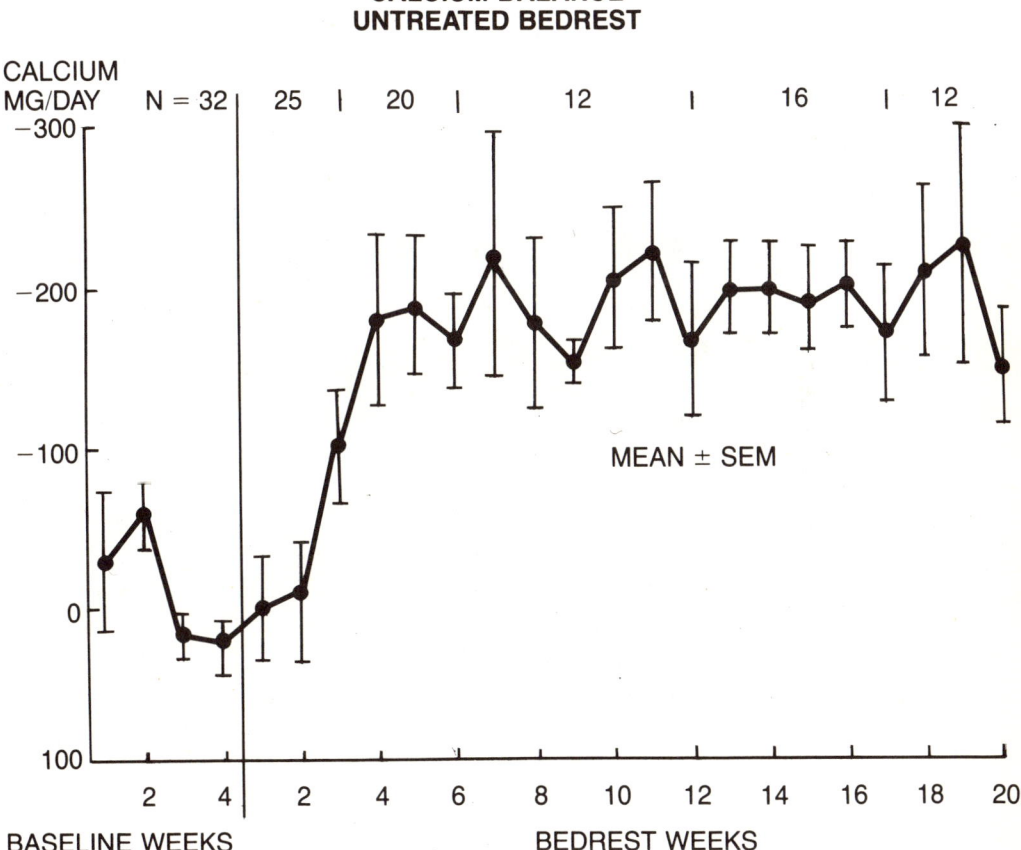

Figure 2. Effect of prolonged bed rest on calcium balance in normal male subjects.[3]

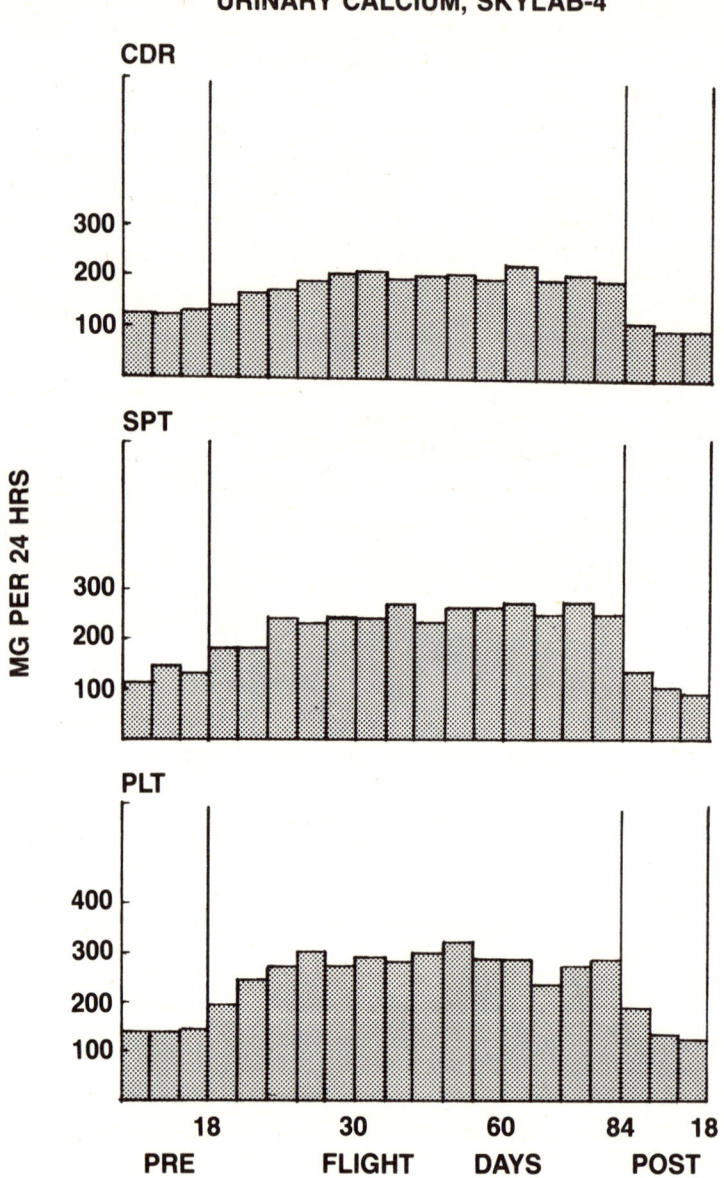

Figure 3. Effect of orbital space flight on urinary calcium excretion in astronauts of the Skylab 84-day flight (SL-4).[4]

Effects of Exercise

Reports have gradually accumulated over the last few years, most of which support the premise that physical activity favors bone formation. Presumably, as Bassett suggested,[6] deforming mechanical stress on bone and cartilage stimulates the activity of osteogenic cells by piezoelectricity. The characteristics of this effect are apparently complex, but the current hypothesis is that the amplitude of generated potential is dependent on the magnitude, frequency and rate of application of the mechanical deforming force. In addition to mechanical forces, however, it is reasonable to assume that physical activity acts through combinations of changes in circulation, neurological stimulation and muscle pull on bone periosteum.

In the recent literature, there are two reviews of the subject.[7,8] Thus far, there apparently are no studies in which subjects or patients are observed and measured first in a state of modest activity and then observed for the effects of a considerable increase in physical activity. The best study to date that supports the premise that physical activity favors bone formation was a comparison by Aloia et al[9] of two groups of postmenopausal women (mean age 53 years and 5.5 years after cessation of menses) who were studied at the same time; one group engaged in exercise classes for one hour, three times a week, for one year. Total body potassium and bone mineral content of the mid-radius showed no significant changes in either group; however, TB Ca decreased over the year by 2.4% in the sedentary control group and increased by 2.6% in the exercise group. The derived calcium balances (change in TB Ca/time in days) were -42 mg/day and +42 mg/day, respectively; the significance of this difference was calculated at $P < 0.001$.

A similar comparative study was made by Smith and Reddan,[10] notable particularly because the mean age of the participants was 82 years. Light to moderate exercise brought about an increase of 4.2% over 36 months in the BMC of the distal one-third of the radius whereas BMC in the control group decreased 2.5% over the same period. The authors concluded that even in the aged, bone may respond with accretion to increased physical stress.

At the other end of the age scale, Emiola and O'Shea[11] divided 45 male and 45 female college students into three groups by level of customary physical activity. Significantly more dense bone was found in the second phalangeal segment of the little finger in the highly active group. Selection of the little finger for bone density measurements in relation to physical activity is curious, but the difference found seems to raise the possibility that physical activity may *in part* exert its action on bone formation through some indirect, humoral factor. Incidentally, the calcium intake levels were similar among three activity groups, but there was an overall significantly positive correlation between calcium intake and bone density.

Three other static group comparisons (by single measurements)—cross-country runners versus age-matched, non-runners,[12] athletes versus controls at several different levels of activity by history,[13] and marathon runners versus age-matched, non-runners[14]—revealed expected differences in bone "density". Norwegian lumbermen at all ages had greater thickness of their metacarpal cortices than less active individuals as reported in other publications,[15] and American tennis players had more dense (BMC) radii and thicker cortices of the humeri in their playing arms than in their non-playing arms.[16,17] The relationship of exercise to bone mass is not entirely simple and direct as indicated by a cross-sectional and longitudinal study of the effects of aging[18]; the rate of bone loss appeared to slow with increasing age (past approximately 60 years) despite gradually decreasing physical activity.

Interrelations of Bone and Muscle

Some investigators have manifested interest in the relationship between muscle and bone mass in response to physical activity. In rats run for four miles a day for 120 days, Donaldson[19] observed a 4% to 7% increase (greater in female rats than in male) in the weight of the leg bones and a corresponding increase in weight of the leg muscles. More recently, Saville and Whyte[20] compared running rats (2000 meters per day) with non-running rats and found that the bone calcium content in the hind legs of the running rats increased in association with an increase in muscle mass, the relationship between muscle mass and bone calcium remaining constant in all animals.

In post-mortem studies of human beings, Doyle et al[21] noted a significant positive correlation between the ash weight of the third lumbar vertebra and the weight of the left psoas muscle and proposed that the weight of a muscle reflects the forces it exerts on bones to which it is attached. Additionally, it was believed that muscle weight is an important determinant of bone mass. In this careful pathological study, the decrease in ash weight of L-3 with age was measured at -8% per decade, similar to that found by Bartley and Arnold.[22] When Ellis et al[23] worked out a predictive formula for whole body potassium based on weight and height (TBK, by whole body counting), unfortunately, they were apparently not yet ready to do TB Ca. They assumed such a relationship, however, from the fact that among the many kinds of patients in whom TBK was measured, the lowest values were observed in patients with disuse osteoporosis. Not all studies, however, confirm a positive muscle mass/bone mass relationship; Sinaki et al[24] found "little correlation" in comparing photon absorption at mid-radius with muscle strength of grip and elbow flexion.

Attempts to Reverse Bone Loss by Exercise

Efforts have been made to determine whether increased physical activity or exercise will counter the loss of bone occurring with either age or inactivity. While the group comparison studies of Aloia et al[9] and of Smith and Reddan[10] are related, only one investigative group has systematically measured the effects of various efforts to reverse the calcium and bone losses associated with inactivity in the same individuals. In bed rest research (at the Public Health

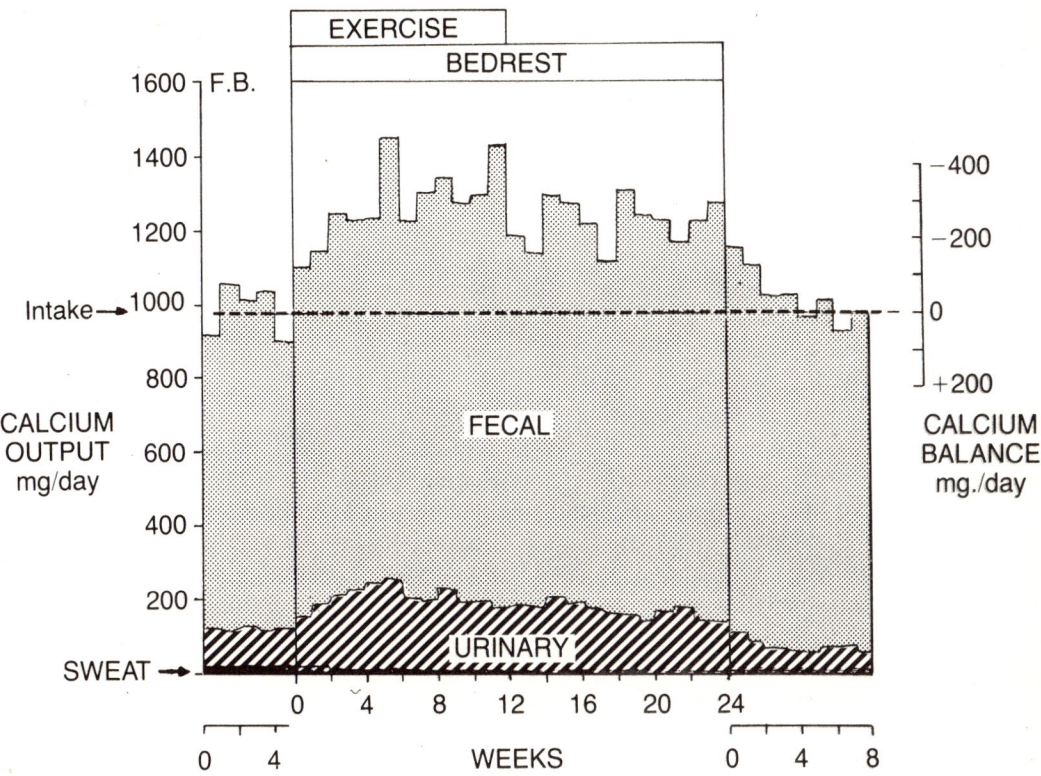

Figure 4. Lack of effect of exercise against resistance on the hypercalciuria and negative calcium balance in a normal male subject during prolonged bed rest.[25]

Service Hospital in San Francisco) sponsored by the National Aeronautics and Space Administration, attempts have been made to develop ways which would protect astronauts' skeletons in future long duration space flights. The effects have been tested of static and intermittent compression (by strong, wide spring bands around shoulders to feet), of intermittent weight-loading (against the bottoms of the feet) and of exercises in bed with and without resistance (Figure 4).[25,26] None of these measures had more than suggestive effects upon either measured calcium metabolic balances or upon density of the os calcis. In an effort to determine how strong an equivalent measure to weight-bearing activity would have to be devised for long-term weightless astronauts, the PHS investigators found that three hours a day quiet standing had a partial effect, while four hours a day of ambulation would prevent loss of mineral, even though the remaining 20 hours a day were spent in bed.

In an uncontrolled effort to seize the immediate opportunity to try to deal with the problem, astronauts during the last Skylab space flight (SL-4, 86 days) used heel-raising exercises against resistance and a simplistic form of "treadmill" devised by an associate engineer-astronaut. The decrease in leg muscle mass, measured at the end of the flight, was significantly less than that observed in the two prior Skylab flights, but data on urinary calcium (Figure 3), calcium balance and os calcis density gave no indication of any impact on hypercalciuria or bone loss. The conclusion thus far reached from these space flights and related bed rest studies, is that the exercise or physical activity which acts to preserve, let alone increase, skeletal mass must be mainly gravitational in character and probably involves several various physiological factors involved in standing and walking.

Effects of Nutrition on Bone Mass

While the number of observations and studies on the relationship of various nutritional factors to bone and mineral metabolism is considerable, there are very few which have involved the actual determination of bone mass. We are mainly dependent, then, on studied effects on urinary calcium, on calcium balance or on calcium kinetics. Space in this mini-review permits mention of only a few principal factors.

Much attention has been directed in recent years to the phenomenon of increases in urinary calcium in response to increases in dietary protein intake[27-29]; this observation has led nutritionists to fear the effects of the national trend toward higher protein intakes on skeletal health. More recently, however, the studies of Spencer et al[30] indicated little change in the urinary level of calcium if the main source of added protein is meat. Spencer attributes this effect to the high phosphate content of meat, since phosphate has a suppressive effect on urinary calcium. Thus, it appears that if Spencer's findings are substantiated, a high meat intake with respect to calcium loss may be less serious than presumed.

The effect of phosphate to suppress urinary excretion of calcium was used by the PHS-San Francisco group to test the effect of phosphate on the negative calcium balance of individuals during prolonged bed rest.[31] While there was full suppression of the hypercalciuria associated with bed rest, fecal calcium tended to increase; thus, the total calcium balance was not favorably affected.

The effects of vitamin D in relation to bone have been extensively studied and characterized. Among its several physiological actions, the role of vitamin D in the intestinal absorption of calcium is best known; its direct action on bone to facilitate mobilization of calcium is less well remembered. Although manifestation of vitamin D deficiency by rickets and osteomalacia was established long ago, recent studies suggest that in elderly and osteoporotic individuals, there may be an impairment of conversion of 25, hydroxyvitamin D to 1,25[32] and/or deficient secretory reserves of 1,25 $(OH)_2D$.[33] Either of these altered processes may explain the inability of older osteoporotic patients to adapt to the low-calcium diets common in this age group.[34]

Relationship of Calcium Intake to Bone Mass

The possible association of low calcium intakes and of impaired intestinal absorption of calcium to calcium balance and bone mass in the human adult was long suppressed, if not denied, in nutrition expert circles. The essential importance of calcium for growth of the skeleton, however, is accepted by pediatricians and the relationship of calcium intake to bone mass at all ages is known to animal experimentalists. One of the earliest studies of the relationship of calcium intake to bone mass (Figure 5) is that of Bauer et al[35] who showed striking responses in trabecular bone in adult cats, both increases and decreases, to manipulations of calcium intake.

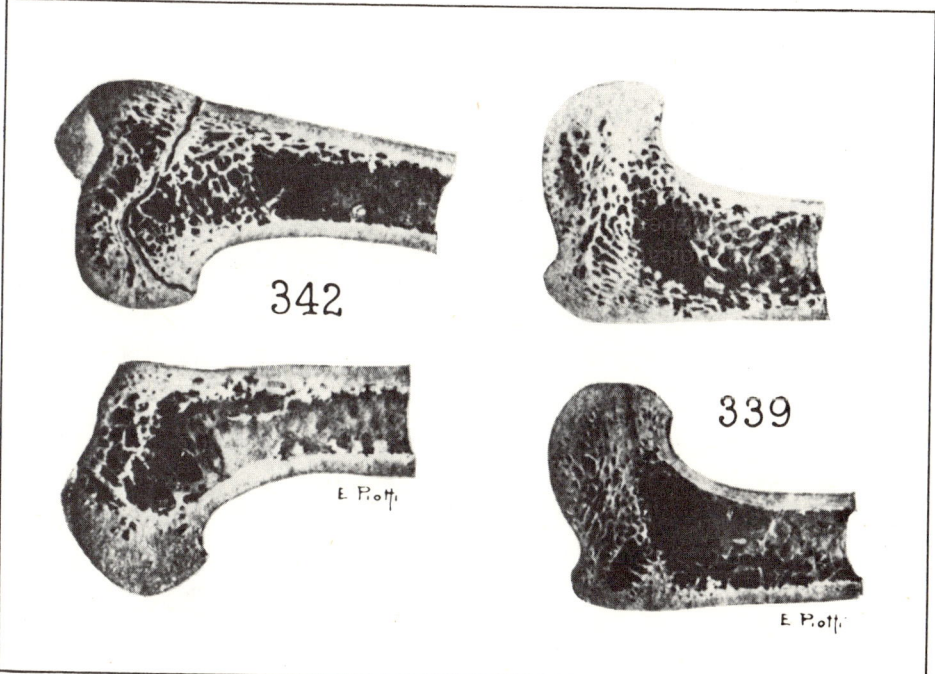

Figure 5. The effect of changes in dietary calcium intake on the amount of cancellous bone in the humeri of adult cats.[35]
In each pair of humeri, the upper bone represents the effect of high calcium intake over several months and the lower bone the effect of low calcium intake over a similar period of time. In cat 342, high calcium intake was given first, followed by low calcium; in cat 339, low calcium intake was given first, followed by high calcium. (Reproduced from the *J Exp Med*[35] by copyright permission of The Rockefeller University Press.)

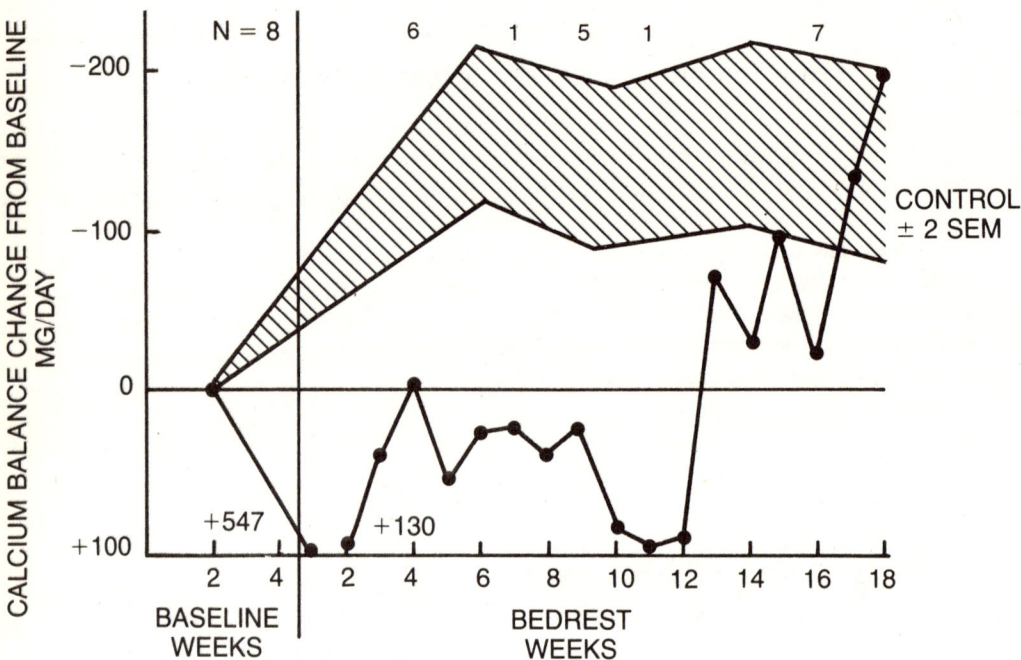

Figure 6. Effect of addition of calcium and phosphate to the dietary intake of normal male subjects during prolonged bed rest.[26]

In human beings, the direct general relationship of calcium intake to balance is known for both children and adults. For many years, the National Research Council Recommended Dietary Allowance (RDA) for calcium, the amount of intake which should ensure meeting the needs of the majority of US population, has been held at 800 mg per day, despite various efforts to raise or lower that level. A particularly pertinent recent study, however, is that of Heaney et al[36] who found mean zero balance at a calcium intake of 990 mg in premenopausal women (mean age, 42 years) and estrogen-replete women (mean age, 47 years). A protective Allowance would have to be substantially higher than the requirement figure determined in this study.

Epidemiologic studies have yielded various results on the relation of customary dietary calcium intake to bone density, but a recent study[37] showed an association between low calcium intake and higher fracture rates at all ages.

More pertinent, however, are two intervention studies in which control groups were compared for changes in BMC of the radius with individuals of similar age and physical activity who were given 750 mg calcium and 400 IU of vitamin D.[38,39] Over a period of three years, the control groups showed significant decreases in BMC, whereas the "treated" groups showed slight, but significant, increases.

Avioli et al[40] and Ireland et al[41] found a gradual decrease in the intestinal absorption of calcium with age. As previously mentioned in relation to vitamin D, this phenomenon may have a pertinent relationship to the multiple etiology of osteoporosis, which will be reviewed in a later chapter by Heaney.[42]

Interrelations of Activity and Nutrition

The only studies that bear directly on the matter of interrelation of physical activity and nutrition are those of the PHS-San Francisco group in their efforts to find a way to stem the outflow of calcium from the skeleton under the influence of the weightlessness model of bed rest. Their earlier observations had shown a protective effect of calcium and phosphorus added to diet during the two months that these elements were given. They later studied the effect of adding 1.2 gm Ca and 1.3 gm P to the regular metabolic diet for four months[26] and found (Figure 6) that during 12 weeks of bed rest, calcium balance was held positive; thereafter, the balance became negative in association with reduced intestinal absorption of calcium. Studies to determine the effects of combined physical exercise and increased mineral dietary intake have not yet been done.

Comment

From a review principally of recent research, both high dietary calcium intake and physical exercise *individually* have positive effects on bone mass. In chronic or relatively acute states of declining bone mass, they act principally to slow net loss of mineral from bone. In the normal, ambulatory animal or human being, various studies indicate that physical exercise, probably in relation to the degree thereof, will *add* some bone mass. The mechanisms of action of the two forces appear to be different: added calcium intake suppresses bone resorption, whereas increased physical activity seems to enhance bone formation or accretion. Normally, the two processes, resorption and formation, are fairly closely coupled. Minor degrees of uncoupling, however, through particular manipulative efforts, may, over time, bring about significant changes in bone mass. Since the mode of action of these two forces is quite different, one would assume that the effects of physical exercise and mineral nutrition together would be additive, at least to a considerable extent. This will not be established as fact until such studies are performed.

In stating that physical exercise is effective, it is important to consider the form of exercise. From the PHS-San Francisco studies, it is apparent that ordinary calisthenics, however valuable they are for maintaining mobility of joints by stretching, do not have much effect, if any, on bone mass. The majority of studies reviewed indicates that effective exercise must be gravitational, ie, involve active weight-bearing movement (as in walking or jogging) or at least must require very vigorous muscle pull on bone.

As a practical recommendation for preservation of skeletal mass, ie, to suppress or slow age-related bone loss, both procedures seem merited. Although there is little evidence of their interrelation, the investigative data, to date, indicates (in the case of added calcium intake) or strongly suggests (in the case of physical exercise) that each is effective.

References

1. Deitrick JE, Whedon GD, Shorr E: Effects of immobilization upon various metabolic and physiologic functions of normal men. *Am J Med* 4:3–36, 1948.
2. Whedon GD, Shorr E: Metabolic studies in paralytic acute anterior poliomyelitis. II. Alterations in calcium and phosphorus metabolism. *J Clin Invest* 36:966–981, 1957.
3. Donaldson CL, Hulley SB, Vogel JM, et al: Effect of prolonged bed rest on bone mineral. *Metabolism* 19:1071–1084, 1970.
4. Whedon GD, Lutwak, L, Reid J, et al: Mineral and nitrogen metabolic studies on Skylab orbital space flights. *Trans Assoc Am Physicians* 87:95–110, 1974.
5. Vogel JM, Whittle MW: Bone mineral content changes in the Skylab astronauts. *Am J Roentgenol, Radium Ther, Nuclear Med* 126:1296–1297, 1976.
6. Bassett CAL, Becker RO: Generation of electric potentials by bone in response to mechanical stress. *Science* 137:1063–1064, 1962.
7. Falch JA: Effect of physical activity on the skeleton. *Tidsskr Nor Laegeforen* 12B, 100:758–761, 1980.
8. Aloia JF: Exercise and skeletal health. *J Am Geriatr Soc* 29:104–107, 1981.
9. Aloia JF, Cohn SH, Ostuni JA, et al: Prevention of involutional bone loss by exercise. *Ann Intern Med* 89:356–358, 1978.
10. Smith EL, Reddan W: Physical activity—a modality for bone accretion in the aged. *Am J Roentgenol, Radium Ther, Nuclear Med* 126:1297, 1976.
11. Emiola L, O'Shea JP: Effect of physical activity and nutrition on bone density measured by radiographic techniques. *Nutrition Reports Int* 17:669–681, 1978.
12. Dalen N, Olsson KE: Bone mineral content and physical activity. *Acta Orthop Scand* 45:170–174, 1974.
13. Nilsson B, Westlin NE: Bone density in athletes. *Clin Orthop* 77:179–182, 1971.
14. Aloia JF, Cohn SH, Babu T, et al: Skeletal mass and body composition in marathon runners. *Metabolism* 27:1793–1796, 1978.
15. Skrobak-Kaczinski J, Andersen KL: Age dependent osteoporosis among men habituated to a high level of physical activity. *Acta Morphol Neerl-Scand* 12:283–292, 1974.
16. Jones HH, Priest JD, Hayes WC, et al: Humeral hypertrophy in response to exercise. *J Bone and Joint Surg* 59–A:204–208, 1977.
17. Huddleston AL, Rockwell D, Kulund DN, et al: Bone mass in lifetime tennis athletes. *JAMA* 244:1107–1109, 1980.
18. Smith DM, Khairi MRA, Norton J, et al: Age and activity effects on rate of bone mineral loss. *J Clin Invest* 58:716–721, 1976.
19. Donaldson HH: Summary of data for the effects of exercise on the organ weights of the albino rat: comparison with similar data from the dog. *Am J Anat* 56:57–70, 1935.
20. Saville PD, Whyte MP: Muscle and bone hypertrophy: positive effect of running exercise in the rat. *Clin Orthop* 65:81–88, 1969.
21. Doyle F, Brown J, LaChance C: Relation between bone mass and muscle weight. *Lancet* 1:391–393, 1970.
22. Bartley MH, Arnold JS: Sex differences in human skeletal involution. *Nature* 214:908–909, 1967.
23. Ellis KJ, Shukla KJ, Cohn SH, et al: A predictor for total body potassium in man based on height, weight, sex and age: applications in metabolic disorders. *J Lab Clin Med* 83:716–727, 1974.

24. Sinaki M, Opitz JL, Wahner HW: Bone mineral content: relationship to muscle strength in normal subjects. *Arch Phys Med Rehabil* 55:508–512, 1974.

25. Hantman DA, Vogel JM, Donaldson CL, et al: Attempts to prevent disuse osteoporosis by treatment with calcitonin, longitudinal compression, and supplementary calcium and phosphate. *J Clin Endocrinol Metab* 36:845–858, 1973.

26. Schneider V: Effect of calcium and phosphorus supplements on bone mineral loss during prolonged bed rest. NASA Technical Report T–81070, 1974.

27. Margen S, Calloway DH: Effect of high protein intake on urinary calcium, magnesium and phosphorus. *Fed Proc* 27:726, 1968.

28. Johnson NE, Alcantara EN, Linkswiler H: Effect of level of protein intake on urinary and fecal calcium and calcium retention of young adult males. *J Nutr* 100:1425–1430, 1970.

29. Bell RR, Engelmann DT, Sie T, et al: Effect of high protein intake on calcium metabolism in the rat. *J Nutr* 105:475–483, 1975.

30. Spencer H, Kramer L, Osis D, et al: Effect of a high protein (meat) intake on calcium metabolism in man. *Am J Clin Nutr* 31:2167–2180, 1978.

31. Hulley SB, Vogel JM, Donaldson CL, et al: The effect of supplemental oral phosphate on the bone mineral changes during prolonged bed rest. *J Clin Invest* 50:2506–2518, 1971.

32. Gallagher JC, Riggs BL, Eisman J, et al: Intestinal calcium absorption and serum vitamin D metabolites in normal subjects and osteoporotic patients: effect of age and dietary calcium. *J Clin Invest* 64:729–736, 1979.

33. Slovik DM, Adams JS, Neer RM, et al: Deficient production of 1,25-dihydroxy vitamin D in elderly osteoporotic patients. *N Engl J Med* 305:372–374, 1981.

34. Whedon GD: Osteoporosis. *N Engl J Med* 305:397–398, 1981.

35. Bauer W, Aub JC, Albright F: A Study of the bone trabeculae as a readily available reserve supply of calcium. *J Exp Med* 49:145, 1929.

36. Heaney RP, Recker RR, Saville PD: Menopausal changes in calcium balance performance. *J Lab Clin Med* 92:953–963, 1978.

37. Matkovic V, Kostial K, Simonovic I, et al: Bone status and fracture rates in two regions of Yugoslavia. *Am J Clin Nutr* 32:540–549, 1979.

38. Smith EL Jr, Reddan W, Smith PE: Physical activity and calcium modalities for bone mineral increase in aged women. *Med Sci Sports Exer* 13:60–64, 1981.

39. Lee CJ, Lawler GS, Johnson GH: Effects of supplementation of the diets with calcium and calcium-rich foods on bone density of elderly females with osteoporosis. *Am J Clin Nutr* 34:819–823, 1981.

40. Avioli LV, McDonald JE, Lee SW: The influence of age on the intestinal absorption of calcium in women and its relation to calcium absorption in postmenopausal osteoporosis. *J Clin Invest* 44:1960–1967, 1965.

41. Ireland P, Fordtran JS: Effect of dietary calcium and age on jejunal calcium absorption in humans studied by intestinal perfusion. *J Clin Invest* 52:2672–2681, 1973.

42. Heaney RP: The role of diet and activity in the treatment of osteoporosis, in White PLW, Mondeika TM (eds): *Diet and Exercise: Synergism in Health Maintenance.* Chicago, American Medical Association, 1982, pp 153–159.

RX: DIET AND ACTIVITY

Moderator: C. Wayne Callaway, MD
Director, Nutrition Consulting Services
Director, Lipid Clinic
Mayo Clinic
Rochester, Minnesota

ENERGY IMBALANCE AND HYPERTENSION RISK†

Ralph S. Paffenbarger, Jr., MD, DrPH*

A balance between energy intake (diet) and energy output (basal metabolism plus exercise) will maintain body weight at a constant level. The demands of vigorous and prolonged physical activity may lead to energy output that is greater than energy intake, resulting in loss of body weight. Conversely, energy output that is less than energy intake will produce a gain in body weight. However, there are other important considerations that need to be recognized, especially in relation to aging and disease.

Physical activity or exercise not only burns up energy but also builds muscle tissue. Unlike fat, muscle tissues use energy even when at rest because of their demands on the metabolic process.[1] Muscle tissues decrease with lack of exercise; the energy requirements of the body at rest or even in ordinary daily activities are also decreased. On the other hand, the appetite and daily energy intake may not decrease, resulting in an imbalance of energy consumption and output. In the absence of sufficient exercise, the excess calories are stored as body fat resulting in obesity.

With advancing age, if individuals become less active or reduce their level of physical activity, adverse effects on bodily health that are often ascribed to the aging process may, in fact, be due to the energy imbalance. Elderly persons who become inactive may incur a loss of weight due to a loss of muscle tissues instead of fat; therefore, many important body functions carried on by the skeletal muscles are gradually impaired.

Obesity in middle-aged persons is most likely due to an energy imbalance caused by a maladjustment of diet in relation to physical activity. Even without computations of energy intake, it is possible to observe this situation in a study population by an assessment of body mass and a change in individual mass with time.

Both gain in body weight and obesity are strong indicators of higher levels of blood pressure and increased risk of hypertension.[2-6] In contrast, vigorous and prolonged physical activity are associated with decreased blood pressure levels and decreased risk of hypertension.[7-10] Using body mass, change in body mass with time, and vigorous sports activity as indices of energy intake and energy output, the key roles of diet and exercise are of demonstrated importance in the prevention and treatment of hypertension.

In an ongoing study of individual characteristics and chronic disease risk in a large population of former college students, the relationships of obesity and lack

---

*Stanford University School of Medicine, Stanford, California
†Report No. XXIII in a series on chronic disease in former college students.

of physical exercise to risk of developing hypertension were investigated. The epidemiologic findings reported in this paper have implications for both dietary and exercise approaches to the control of obesity and hypertension.

Materials and Methods

Two data bases were available for study:

1) 7,685 normotensive men who attended the University of Pennsylvania between 1931 and 1940 were followed for 22–31 years, from the time of college record to 1962, for the occurrence of hypertension.[11]

2) 14,998 normotensive men who entered Harvard University between 1916 and 1950 were followed for six to ten years, 1962 or 1966 to 1972, for the occurrence of hypertension.[8,10]

In the University of Pennsylvania study, only men less than 30 years of age at time of college physical examination were included. Incidence rates of hypertension, computed for the number of subjects at risk (7,685) were adjusted by the indirect method for differences in student age (five-year groups) and follow-up intervals (five-year groups). Relative risks represented the risk of developing hypertension among former students with a given characteristic as compared with the risk among their counterparts without that characteristic. Attributable risks (clinical) were computed as $1 - \frac{1}{\text{relative risk}} \times 100$; attributable risks (community) as $\frac{(\text{prevalence of characteristic}) \times (\text{relative risk} - 1)}{1 + (\text{prevalence of characteristic}) \times (\text{relative risk} - 1)} \times 100$.

Clinical and community attributable risks for a given student characteristic were adjusted only for differences in age and follow-up interval. Frequency distributions of characteristics to be quantified were separated where possible into the quartile or half of former students at higher or lower risk of hypertension.

In the Harvard University study, for first-order estimates of the incidence of hypertension, rates were adjusted for differences in alumnus age using the indirect method and five-year age groups by man-years of observation for the total population (105,662 man-years) as standard. Multivariate estimates of the incidence of hypertension, relative risks, and attributable risks (clinical) were based on a logistic model, using maximum likelihood estimates[12] related to vigorous sports play, by levels of body mass index and weight gain since college, being adjusted for other alumnus characteristics known to alter incidence (eg, age and parental history of hypertension). Attributable risks (community) of hypertension for individual alumnus characteristics were computed as described earlier in the University of Pennsylvania study.

Significant probabilities in both sets of data were based on adjusted rates, using as standard the total population (former students or man-years of follow-up) of any two groups being compared. All probability (P) values cited are for a two-tailed test.

Results

In the 22–31 years between physical examinations at the University of Pennsylvania and questionnaire response in 1962, 671 (9%) of 7,685 respondents had developed hypertension (diagnosed by a physician). These men ranged from 20 to 60 years of age at the time of diagnosis. Age- and interval-adjusted incidence rates of hypertension, as related to the presence or absence of selected student characteristics, were computed as were relative risks of hypertension from less participation in sports, greater body mass, higher levels of blood pressure, and history of parental hypertension (Table 1).

Table 1. Relative and Attributable Risks of Hypertension among University of Pennsylvania Alumni in a 22–31 Year Follow-up since College, by Student Characteristics

Student Characteristic	Prevalence of Characteristic, %	Relative Risk of Hypertension* ± 1 S.E.	P	Clinical Attributable Risk Estimate %
Sports play <5 hr/week	43.5	1.32 ± 0.13	0.004	24.2
Ponderal index† <12.9 units	25.6	1.34 ± 0.11	<0.001	25.4
Systolic blood pressure 130+ mm Hg	24.2	2.72 ± 0.21	<0.001	63.2
Parental hypertension present	8.7	1.70 ± 0.18	0.002	41.2

*Adjusted for differences in age and follow-up interval.
†Height in inches over cube root of weight in pounds.

The students (43.5%) who reported that they participated in intramural sports less than five hours per week, or not at all, experienced a higher age- and interval-adjusted incidence rate of hypertension (13.9%) then did their more active classmates (8.2%), a 32% increased risk for the less active. Comparable findings, not tabulated, were observed with regard to participation in intercollegiate athletics. Adjusted incidence rates were 9.1% for non-athletes as compared with 7.4% for the 19.7% of students who were varsity athletes, a relative risk of 1.29 for non-athletes.

Interval incidence rates were computed by measures of ponderal index (height in inches/$\sqrt[3]{\text{weight in pounds}}$) at the time of college physical examination. The rates showed a steady increase in risk of developing hypertension as body mass increased. At the breakpoint of <12.9 units, representing one-quarter of the students, the rates were 10.6% for the heavier men as compared with 7.9% for those who were more lean, a relative risk of 1.34 for the former group.

Findings ran parallel when incidence of hypertension was computed in terms of height-specific and height-adjusted body weight. Height-adjusted mean weights for students who developed hypertension in the follow-up interval were 68.4 ± 10.5 kg (150.9 ± 23.1 lbs) and for their normotensive classmates, 66.6 ± 9.2 kg (146.8 ± 20.2 lbs).

Student blood pressure levels and parental histories of hypertension were the strongest predictors of hypertension risk in middle life and, accordingly, are considered in conjunction with body weight and exercise levels for their relative contributions to risk.

Both systolic and diastolic blood pressure levels in college students were associated with the incidence of hypertension in the 22–31 year follow-up, ending in 1962. The higher the blood pressure level in college students, the higher the incidence of subsequent hypertension. Interval incidence rates for the quartile of students with systolic levels of 130+ mm Hg were more than one and one-half times that of the remainder of students, 16.6% and 6.1% respectively. Corresponding rates for diastolic levels (not tabulated) at a breakpoint of 80+ mm Hg, which identified one-quarter of the students, were 14.3% and 6.6%, a relative risk of 2.17. At the time of college physical examination, the students (8.7%) who reported one or both parents hypertensive, were at higher risk of becoming hypertensive themselves (13.9%) than were students whose parents were not hypertensive (8.2%), a 70% excess risk.

Table 1 shows the proportion of students with clinical attributable risks who became hypertensive during the follow-up interval, but might have been expected to remain normotensive had they not manifested these characteristics. These attributable risk estimates are theoretical and assume: that there is an etiologic relationship between each characteristic and hypertension; that the presence or absence of the characteristics remains constant over the follow-up interval; that dose-effect responses exist; that the characteristics could be altered from higher to lower risk levels; and that other influences on the incidence of hypertension are distributed similarly in students with high and low levels of the risk-characteristics. The estimates might be considered as theoretical assessments of the effect of treating hypertension among the afflicted. An average reduction in risk was estimated for each changed characteristic after discounting the effect of age and follow-up interval. As seen, the incidence of hypertension in the physically less active students would have been lowered by 24.2% if they had been more active. If overweight students had remained lean (with a ponderal index of 12.9+ units), their risk would have been reduced by 25.4%. The risks attributed to higher levels of systolic blood pressure and the presence of parental hypertension were 63.2% and 41.2%, respectively.

Community attributable risks, which take the prevalence of the characteristics into consideration, are the estimated reductions in hypertension incidence in the total population of 7,685 former students that might have occurred if each of these risk characteristics had not existed. Such estimates might be construed as the effects of treating hypertension within a population. The estimated reduction in incidence rates might have been for: reduced sports play, 12.2%, obesity 8.0%, elevated systolic blood pressure, 29.6%, and parental hypertension, 5.7%.

The indices of energy output and energy intake, ie, vigorous sports play and ponderal index, clearly identify those students at altered risk of hypertension. Presumably, one could also identify those whose hypertension would come under control through judicious personal action, ie, increase in physical activity and decrease in body weight through participation in vigorous exercise and restriction of energy intake.

In the Harvard University study of 14,998 alumni (aged 35–74 years) who reported themselves free of physician-diagnosed hypertension in 1962 or 1966, 681 (4.5%) developed hypertension by 1972. Age-adjusted incidence rates and relative risks of hypertension were computed for absence of vigorous sports play, greater body mass, body mass index gain since college, and history of parental hypertension (Table 2). Measures of energy expenditure were limited to

Table 2. Relative and Attributable Risks of Hypertension among Harvard University Alumni in a 6–10 Year Follow-up, 1962 or 1966-1972, by Alumnus Characteristics

Alumnus Characteristic	Prevalence of Characteristic, %	Relative Risk of Hypertension* ± 1 S.E.	P	Clinical Attributable Risk Estimate %
No vigorous sports play†	65.0	1.52 ± 0.17	<0.001	34.2
Body mass index‡ 36+ units	36.3	1.43 ± 0.15	<0.001	30.0
Body mass index gain since college 5+ units	40.8	1.44 ± 0.15	<0.001	30.7
Parental hypertension present	38.8	1.91 ± 0.18	<0.001	47.6

*Adjusted for differences in age, follow-up interval, and each of the other characteristics listed.
†Activities requiring 7.5 kilocalories or more per minute to perform.
‡Quetelet's index of weight in pounds over height in inches squared times 1000.

vigorous sports play since it had been shown previously that activities not requiring bursts of energy output, eg, stair climbing, walking and light sports play, did not influence risk of hypertension in this population.[8,10] Vigorous sports were defined as those activities requiring 7.5+ kcal per minute of energy output to perform and, they generally represented swimming and running activities, including casual and competitive field and court sports. The relative risks displayed were adjusted for age, follow-up interval, and each of the other characteristics listed.

The alumni (65.0%) who did not participate in vigorous sports in 1962 or 1966 were at 52% increased risk of developing hypertension in the six to ten year follow-up interval compared with those who participated in such sports.

Interval incidence rates were computed by measures of body mass (Quetelet's index of weight in pounds/height in inches squared × 1000) at time of first questionnaire response (1962 or 1966). These rates showed a steady increase in hypertension with increasing body mass. The breakpoint of 36+ units, which identifies men 20% or more over "ideal" weight for height,[13] identified 36.3% of the alumni and a 43% increased risk of hypertension over men who were of lower weight.

Men who had gained in excess of five units of body mass since college, an interval that ranged from 16 to 50 years, comprised 40.8% of the total. This gain in body weight, 11.3+ kg (25+ pounds), represents acquisition of excess body fat and was associated with a 44% increased risk of hypertension over that for a lesser gain.

Again, parental history of hypertension, representing more than 25,000 people (many of whom had died), was related to risk of hypertension in Harvard men. The alumni who reported one or both parents hypertensive (38.8%) were at nearly twice the risk of becoming hypertensive (91% increase) as were alumni with normotensive parents.

Table 2 gives clinical attributable risks for alumnus characteristics in the Harvard University study applying the same theoretical assumptions as described for the University of Pennsylvania study (cause-and-effect, persistance of characteristics, proportional changes, risk-characteristics alterability, and equivalent distributions of other risk characteristics). Other factors being equal, the incidence of hypertension might have been reduced by 30% to 50% if the less vigorous alumni had been more active, the overweight more lean, the weight gainers had gained less than 11.3 kg, and if instead of hypertensive parents, alumni had normotensive parents. Combinations of these characteristics further increased the risk.[10]

Table 3 presents a similar analysis for the three characteristics associated with the issue of energy intake and energy output in hypertension control, namely, vigorous sports play, body mass, and body mass gain. Age and parental history of hypertension, one of the strongest risk characteristics, are also considered. An average reduction in risk is estimated for each unit change in a given characteris-

Table 3. Relative and Attributable Risks of Hypertension among Harvard University Alumni in a 6–10 Year Follow-up, 1962 or 1966-1972, with change in Alumnus Characteristics

Alumnus Characteristic	Unit change in Characteristic	Relative Risk of Hypertension per Unit Change* ± 1 S.E.	P	Clinical Attributable Risk Estimate %
Vigorous sports play†	Increase 1 hr/wk	0.95 ± 0.02	0.029	5.1
Body mass index‡	Decrease 1 unit	0.92 ± 0.01	<0.001	7.9
Body mass index change	Decrease 1 unit	0.98 ± 0.02	0.116	2.2

*Adjusted for differences in age, parental history of hypertension, follow-up interval, and each of the other characteristics listed.
†Activities requiring 7.5 kilocalories or more per minute to perform.
‡Quetelet's index of weight in pounds over height in inches squared times 1000.

tic after discounting the effects of age, parental history, follow-up interval, and the other two characteristics listed. Thus, hypertension incidence might have been reduced by 5.1% for each one-hour increase in weekly participation in vigorous sports, or approximately a 25% reduction in risk for an alumnus who increased his vigorous sports participation by five hours per week. A decrease in body mass index of one unit (approximately 2.3 kg or 5 lbs) might have been accompanied by a reduction of 7.9%, or a loss of 9.1 kg (20 lbs), by a lowering of about 30%. The prevention of one body mass index unit of weight gain since college might have been accompanied by a minimal risk lowering of 2.2%; the prevention of four units of weight gain by a modest lowering of 8% or 9%.

Taking the entire population of nearly 15,000 alumni into consideration, the potential reduction in hypertension incidence during the 6 to 10 year follow-up interval might have been 25.3% if all alumni had participated in vigorous sports, 13.5% if all had been less than 11.3 kg (25 lbs) overweight, and 15.2% if all had gained less than 11.3 kg since college. The added risk of hypertension from a combination of excess body mass and nonparticipation in vigorous sports, indices of excess energy intake and deficient energy output, may be estimated to be approximately 50%. The study suggests that a proper prescription of vigorous exercise and prudent diet may effectively "treat" half of the hypertensives in such populations.

Figure 1 gives age-adjusted incidence rates and relative risks of hypertension for alumni classified by vigorous sports play, body mass index (<36 or 36+ units), and body mass index gain since college (<5 or 5+ units). The pairs of bars

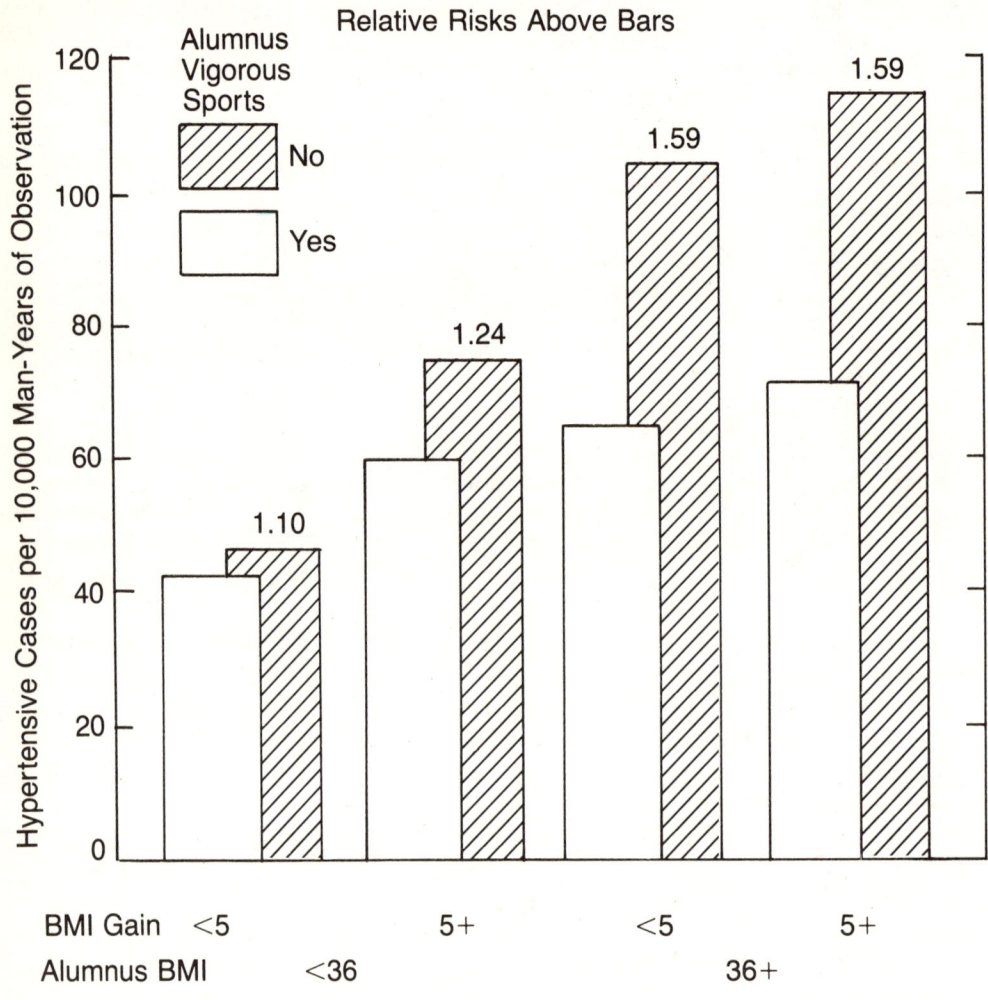

Figure 1. Age-adjusted rates and relative risks of hypertension by combinations of vigorous sports play, alumnus body mass index, and body mass index gain since college.

from left to right in the Figure comprise, respectively, 52%, 20%, 10%, and 18% of the 105,662 man-years of observation. The alumni who were overweight and those who continued to gain weight extensively following their college physical examination were at greater risk of hypertension; the reduced risk of hypertension attached to vigorous activities was substantial only for those with increased weight-for-height. As compared with more active men of their size, alumni who were 11.3+ kg over "ideal" weight and not participating in vigorous sports had a 59% increased risk of hypertension in the six to ten year follow-up.

Discussion

Direct evidence on the effect of dietary and exercise regimens in the treatment of hypertension is not currently available from epidemiologic studies. Future ventures must search for simplified methods of assessing such regimens, together with appropriate indices of these regimens (total body mass; lean mass, fat mass; and type, frequency, timing, duration, and intensity of physical activities). Such explorations must determine the effect of interactions among these variables with respect to the incidence of hypertension and its sequelae (heart, brain, and kidney disease) and to longevity *per se*.

Meanwhile, the data reported here indicate the relationships of increased body mass and lack of participation in vigorous sports (indices of energy intake and energy output) to hypertension incidence. Persons who were overweight and the less active were both at increased risk of hypertension; a combination of excess weight and lack of vigorous exercise further increased the risk. Attributable risk estimates, measures of the potential reduction in hypertension incidence from host-characteristic intervention, suggest that failure to balance energy intake and energy output may account for a sizeable fraction of hypertension incidence, in both a clinical and community sense, ie, both individually and *en masse*.

Maintenance of a balanced energy intake and output in hypertension control may require both dietary and exercise regimens. If diet limitations are imposed, care must be taken to provide all necessary nutrients.[14] Salt consumption, long suspected as being linked with hypertension, especially among the genetically predisposed, might best be restricted.[15-19] Control of diet alone, however, even though it may lead to reduced fat stores, is not sufficient. Without adequate physical exercise, diet does not build muscle tissues required for good health. We may presume that most of the college alumni studied had been reasonably well-fed. The results of the present investigation have shown that the importance of vigorous exercise is even greater for the heavier men, at least for prevention of hypertension, and presumably for its effective treatment. The college and alumni data sources do not show which of these men may have been on a prescribed or self-imposed diet, but the details of their energy intake would be unlikely to bias or alter the findings that have been presented here.

Summary

Physical examination and athletic records of former students from the University of Pennsylvania and Harvard University, supplemented with alumni questionnaire data on health and exercise patterns, permitted computation of incidence rates of hypertension in terms of levels of body mass, body mass gain since college, and sports participation. Relative and attributable risks of developing hypertension provided estimates of the roles of diet and exercise in the prevention and control of hypertension. The upper quartile of students by weight-for-height were 34% more likely to become hypertensive than those weighing less. The 40% of the students who spent less than five hours per week playing sports were at 32% increased risk over the more active. The approximately one-third of the alumni who were most overweight-for-height were at 43% increased risk compared with the more slender alumni, and the 40% who had gained 11.3+ kg (25+ lbs) since college were at 44% increased risk over those with lesser gain. The two-thirds of alumni who did not participate in vigorous sports were at 52% increased risk over men who engaged in such sports. Clinical attributable risks for the more overweight, those who had gained an excess of 11.3+ kg, and the less vigorous were 30%, 31%, and 34%, respectively, suggesting that weight control or vigorous activities in middle life would reduce risk by about one-third. A sustained fit and active lifestyle might reduce risk of hypertension by approximately 50%.

Acknowledgment

This work was supported by U.S. Public Health Service research grant HL 24133 from the National Heart, Lung, and Blood Institute.

References

1. Keys A, Taylor HL, Grande F: Basal metabolism and age of adult man. *Metabolism* 22:579–587, 1973.
2. Levy RL, White PD, Stroud WD, et al: Sustained hypertension. Predisposing factors and causes of disability and death. *JAMA* 135:77–80, 1947.
3. Thomas CB: The heritage of hypertension. *Am J Med Sci* 224:367–376, 1952.
4. Tyroler HA, Heyden S, Hames CG: Weight and hypertension: Evans County studies of blacks and whites, in Paul O (ed): *Epidemiology and Control of Hypertension*. New York and London, Stratton Intercontinental Medical Book Corp, 1975, pp 177–204.
5. Stamler J, Berkson DM, Dyer A, et al: Relationship of multiple variables to blood pressure—findings from four Chicago epidemiologic studies, in Paul O (ed): *Epidemiology and Control of Hypertension*. New York and London, Stratton Intercontinental Medical Book Corp, 1975, pp 307–356.
6. Stamler R, Stamler J, Riedlinger MS, et al: Weight and blood pressure findings in hypertension screening of 1 million Americans. *JAMA* 240:1607–1610, 1978.
7. Boyer JL, Kasch FW: Exercise in hypertensive men. *JAMA* 211:1668–1671, 1970.
8. Paffenbarger RS Jr, Wing AL, Hyde RT, et al: Contemporary physical activity and incidence of hypertension in college alumni. Abstracts *Circulation* 1979, 59–60 (Supp II):76.
9. Stamler J, Farinaro E, Mojonnier LM, et al: Prevention and control of hypertension by nutritional-hygienic means: long-term experience of the Chicago Coronary Prevention Evaluation Program. *JAMA* 243:1819–1923, 1980.
10. Paffenbarger RS Jr, Wing AL, Hyde RT, et al: Physical activity and incidence of hypertension in college alumni. Submitted for publication.
11. Paffenbarger RS Jr, Thorne MC, Wing AL: Chronic disease in former college students. VIII. Characteristics in youth predisposing to hypertension in later years. *Am J Epidemiol* 88:25–32, 1968.
12. Cornfield J: Joint dependence of risk of coronary heart disease on serum cholesterol and systolic blood pressure: a discriminant function analysis. *Fed Proc* 21:58–61, 1962.
13. Metropolitan Life Insurance Company: New weight standards for men and women. *Stat Bull Metropol Life Ins Co* 40:1–4 (Nov–Dec) 1959.
14. Åstrand PO: Diet and exercise—how to secure an adequate intake of essential nutrients. *Internat Med* 1:23–26, 1979.
15. Dahl LK, Schackow E: Effects of chronic excess salt ingestion: experimental hypertension in the rat. *Can Med Assoc J* 90:155–160, 1964.
16. Tobian L: Current status of salt in hypertension, in Paul O (ed): *Epidemiology and Control of Hypertension*. New York and London, Stratton Intercontinental Medical Book Corp, 1975, pp 131–146.
17. Freis ED: Salt, volume and the prevention of hypertension. *Circulation* 53:589–595, 1976.
18. Lowering blood pressure without drugs; editorial. *Lancet* 1980, 2:459–461.
19. New evidence linking salt and hypertension; editorial. *Br Med J* 1981, 282:1993–1994.

PHYSICAL ACTIVITY AND DIET IN THE TREATMENT OF CORONARY HEART DISEASE

Samuel M. Fox, III, MD*
James A. Metcalf, PhD**

Until utilization of the automobile became widespread, some physical activity was necessary for almost everyone, even in the technically advanced countries. Automation in the workplace has replaced physically demanding jobs. Television attracts spectators who might otherwise be engaged in more active recreation. Life-styles today may offer little physical activity for many people unless they personally seek an active program.

Parallel to these trends, there was a statistically significant increase in the incidence of coronary deaths from the 1920s through the mid-1960s in inverse proportion to the average citizen's daily expenditure of physical energy. Physical inactivity has been accepted for listing as a coronary "risk factor" by most review groups, although usually considered less influential than cigarette smoking and elevations of blood pressure and serum cholesterol levels. It has been demonstrated that effective management of hypertension[1] and the lowering of serum lipids coupled with some reduction of smoking[2] can reduce the incidence of coronary disease. Similar studies on tobacco use alone may not be considered ethically acceptable since its use is so widely condemned that investigators might reject the concept of a "control group" not being encouraged to stop smoking.

The importance of physical activity was recognized over 2300 years ago in the Greek Academy where its founder, Plato, writes of Timaeus extolling exercise when telling Socrates ". . . and by moderate exercise reduces to order according to their affinities the particles and affections which are wandering about the body . . ." followed by "Wherefore of all modes of purifying and reuniting the body the best is gymnastic."

Until recently, most comparisons of the incidence of coronary disease to physical activity levels were related to occupational groups in which the majority of studies showed an inverse relationship, ie, the greater the physical activity, the less the coronary manifestations and, particularly, the associated coronary mortality. Two studies, however, have recently focused on recreational and free-time activities which are more relevant to what the average citizen, and the attending physician, must consider.

*Georgetown University, Washington, D.C.
**George Mason University, Fairfax, Virginia

Observational Studies

Morris et al obtained a two-day record of activities from over 16,800 male Civil Servants in Britain from 1968–70, along with a completed questionnaire on habits and personal history. The men who were later stricken with a first clinical attack of coronary heart disease (CHD) had reported less than half the previous involvement in "vigorous" exercise (ie, activities likely to reach peaks of energy output of 7½ kcal/min) compared with matched disease-free controls.[3,4] The relative risk of developing coronary disease was reduced by more than 50% in men who engaged in vigorous exercise compared to men who did not; the risk was further reduced in those men who reported increased amounts of vigorous exercise.

Vigorous activities produce a training effect on the cardiovascular system. These activities include active forms of recreation (swimming, tennis), "keep fit" exercises, heavy work (digging, wood sawing and planing) and "getting about quickly" at greater than 4 miles per hour (mph) or over rough country or bicycling faster than 11 mph. Painting, paper hanging, polishing the car, hoeing the garden and cutting hedges, considered to require 4 to 7 kcal/min, did not correlate with a lesser incidence of coronary disease. A time threshold of 30 min appeared to apply before heavy physical work became "beneficial".[3] Overall activity, not including vigorous activity, appeared to provide only a weak associated advantage. The benefit was found among men of all ages (40 to 64 years), though more striking differences were seen in later middle age and early old age. There was also a definable benefit in men with a family history of CHD, cigarette smokers, the obese, those of short stature, and in men with severe hypertension and subclinical angina. Benefit was also observed in those with lesser risk of CHD.

Among over 16,000 Harvard male alumni, Paffenbarger et al[5] found a similar inverse incidence of first heart attacks relative to energy expenditure patterns. "Adult exercise was independent of other influences on heart attack risk, and peak exertion as strenuous sports play enhanced the effect of total energy expenditure.". . . . "Ex-varsity athletes retained lower risk only if they maintained a high physical activity index as alumni." Sports were categorized according to the amount of energy expended, eg, light sports—5 kcal/min, strenuous sports—10 kcal/min, and combinations of the two—7.5 kcal/min. Alumni were classified according to the number of hours per week engaged in light or strenuous sports play. A physical activity index was devised and the equivalent energy output was expressed in kcal/week. Sixty percent of person-years of observation of the alumni were on the low side of 2000 kcal/week and 40% were above 2000 kcal/week. There was a 64% increased risk of heart attack in the less active group as compared to those expending more than 2000 kcal/week.

The men who reported no strenuous sports play were at 38% greater risk of heart attack than those who engaged in strenuous sports. No significant difference was found between those who participated in light sports and those reporting essentially minimal physical activity. Men who played less than three hours per week of strenuous sports (74% of person-years observed) had a 54% higher age-adjusted heart attack rate than men who played strenuous sports three or more hours per week. Physical inactivity and cigarette smoking were tied for second ranking as risk factors behind a history of hypertension, but ahead of body mass index, stature and early parental heart attack. The significance of physical activity was independent of other risk factor status and was found to apply to all age groups from 35 to 74 years. These two studies are remarkably similar with discordance only in relation to sudden death. Among Harvard alumni, no significant inverse relationship of sudden death with habitual levels of previous physical activity was observed while Morris et al[4] found that habitual vigorous activity apparently protected against rapidly fatal heart attacks.

The Framingham study demonstrated a lesser, but significantly diminished, overall mortality due to all forms of cardiovascular disease and ischemic heart disease relative to the overall level of physical activity in men, but not among women.[6] Rosenman observed a 39% lower incidence of coronary events in "Type A" men (time-pressured, hostile, demanding of self) engaged in regular exercise compared to sedentary colleagues, but no difference between activity level groups of "Type B" men in the Western Collaborative Group Study.[7] The influence of personal choice and subtle mechanism effecting physical drive and energy may contribute significantly to differences found in these observational studies. Controlled intervention study designs would help reduce the skepticism related to personal and other factors.

Intervention Studies

Prospective intervention studies, using randomly assigned "healthy" or "high risk" groups, with the predominant intervention being differing levels of physical activity, have been considered but not yet initiated beyond a pilot trial. The problems of compliance and the number of subjects required have been deemed too formidable, but there is a continuing great need to more clearly define the role of increased habitual physical activity in the lives of sedentary Americans.

Of five randomized rehabilitation studies, involving post-myocardial infarction patients, only one has demonstrated a *statistically* significant difference in mortality.[8] The major alterations were lipid level and blood pressure reductions rather than increased physical work capacity or decreased tobacco use. A reduced coronary mortality ($p<.02$) and sudden deaths ($p<.01$) were observed in the intervention group with the major difference being seen within the first six months post-infarction.

An earlier Finnish study,[9] and one in Ontario,[10] revealed no significant difference while the study in Goteborg, Sweden[11] had a 31% favorable outcome, falling short of being statistically significant ($p<.10$). Likewise, an attempt in the United States,[12] compromised by budget reductions, was 37% effective in reducing mortality, but within the numbers available, this was not statistically significant (p<.22). There was a significant reduction in fatal reinfarctions (p<.05).

Mechanisms That May Be Preventive

An increase in habitual physical activity, particularly of the endurance-stimulating type, is likely to produce changes in a number of factors or responses in varying degrees (Table 1). Many of these appear to have the potential for contributing to a preventive program, although conclusive proof of such effect in humans is inadequate. These are reviewed in detail in other publications[13,14] and, thus, those relating to diet and energy balance will be emphasized here.

A recent report of the effects of exercise in monkeys on an atherogenic diet demonstrated ischemic electrocardiographic changes, angiographic signs of coronary artery narrowing, and sudden death only in the non-exercising monkeys in which post-mortem examination revealed marked coronary atherosclerosis and stenoses.[15] "Exercise was associated with substantially reduced overall atherosclerotic involvement, lesion size, and collagen accumulation; it also produced much larger hearts and wider coronary arteries, further reducing the degree of luminal narrowing." Serum total cholesterol was not altered, but significantly higher levels of high-density lipoprotein (HDL) cholesterol and much lower levels of low-density lipoprotein (LDL) triglycerides were observed in the exercise group.

Although atherogenic mechanisms in monkeys may not be similar to those in man, it is possible that similar responses would be found in man. Selvester et al[16] observed that atherosclerotic disease of the coronary arteries progressed less rapidly in post-infarct patients who engaged in physical endurance training than in their less active counterparts. The coronary narrowing and occurrence of new infarctions (over an average of 20 months between angiograms) was less among those with progressively more involvement in physical training. The number of "progressible" vessels (ie, major coronary arteries with 50% or more, but less than 100% narrowing visible on initial angiogram) actually showing progression among participants engaged in a high level of activity was half the rate found in the inactive participants, with a greater effect among smokers than non-smokers.

Although the enjoyment of pleasant activities and the psychological benefits during or after exercise help maintain the involvement of most participants, there is as yet no proof that these factors actually decrease the risk of coronary heart disease. Likewise, it has been difficult to document that the almost predictable increase in cardiovascular work capacity and functional reserves may decrease vulnerability to ischemia or infarction, particularly in association with physical effort. A most encouraging report from Ehsani et al[17] demonstrated less ischemic electrocardiographic abnormalities after 12 months of intense endurance exercise training, at both the same and greater total body work loads and

Table 1. Potential Preventive Benefits resulting from an Increase in Habitual Physical Activity

I. Increased Physiologic Capacity:
Increased physical performance capacity
Lower heart rate at a specific task
Lower blood pressure at a specific task
Lower rate and depth of breathing required
Better air passage and lung function
Greater efficiency and less perceived effort
More appropriate peripheral blood distribution and return
Enhanced blood volume and red cell mass
Less tendency for hemoconcentration
Less tendency for thrombophlebitis and pulmonary emboli
Better heat and cold adaptation and tolerance
Stimulus for increased arterial size
Stimulus for collateral vessels to bypass obstruction
Less rapid loss of bone minerals with age
Stimulus for better cartilage protection of joints
Decreased inappropriate gastric acid secretion
Decreased appetite after exercise (½-hour)
Ability to eat more yet not gain weight
Better bowel function
Improved function and appearance of the skin
Reduced allergic reactions (asthma, hay fever)

II. Biochemical Benefits:
Expanded diet permits greater intake of vitamins, minerals and other desirable dietary elements
Reduction in Low Density Lipoprotein Cholesterol
Increase in High Density Lipoprotein Cholesterol
Reduced Total Serum Cholesterol
Reduced Serum Triglycerides
Increased effectiveness of insulin
Reduced platelet adhesiveness
Increased fibrinolysis (early clot dissolution)
Decreased inappropriate catecholamine (adrenalin) responses to stress
Decreased vulnerability or susceptibility to cardiac dysrhythmia.

III. Psychological Benefits:
Enhanced feelings of energy, enthusiasm and well being—more stamina
Decreased depression
Enhanced self image
Less "strain" resulting from psychic "stress"
Better relaxation and sleep
More satisfactory sexual responses
Less craving for stimulants and tranquilizers

IV. Socio-Economic Benefits:
More optimism, enthusiasm, creativity
Less illness, absenteeism
Shorter illness course and fewer complications
Reduced medical expenses

"double product" of systolic blood pressure multiplied by the heart rate. The double product at which 0.1 mV of ST depression first appeared was 22% greater after training, which should represent an expanded capability for contending with stress at a decreased risk.

Intervention at the biochemical level, with a potentially more direct influence on the basic atherosclerotic-thrombotic process itself, appears to hold great promise for reducing the morbidity and mortality of CHD.

Numerous studies define a higher level of high density lipoprotein (HDL) cholesterol in those men and women who are habitually more active physically.[18] Less consistent has been the ability to demonstrate an increase in HDL-cholesterol and/or an increase of HDL in relation to either total or low density lipoprotein (LDL) cholesterol as a response to physical training.

An increase in HDL-cholesterol is thought to provide benefit by helping to remove atherogenic lipid fractions, LDL-cholesterol in particular, from the serum and arterial wall for transport to the liver, catabolism and excretion.[19] High density lipoproteins may also effectively compete with LDL for arterial wall attachment, without stimulating atherogenesis.[20]

Leon et al[21] observed a 15.6% increase in HDL, and an HDL/LDL ratio increase of 25.9% above pretraining levels among six sedentary obese young men completing 16 weeks of vigorous walking for 90 minutes, five days a week. A decrease in HDL, however, was noted by Allison et al[22] during an eight week program in which the subjects increased their level of exercise to either 30 or 45 minutes of running three times a week; however, a significant increase in aerobic capacity was produced. The HDL increase observed by Leon et al[21] might be attributed to the longer duration of the study with the suggestion that there is a latent period prior to an increase in HDL. Allison et al[22] point out that it may be necessary to have an accompanying decline in triglycerides to initiate or facilitate an HDL increase. This was not seen in the majority of their subjects, but was found in the ten subjects with an HDL increase. The authors reviewed previous studies and pointed toward the need to examine the responses of various HDL subfractions.[22]

Although Allison's exercisers spontaneously increased dietary fat intake, there was no significant change in weight. Leon made no attempt to alter the diet of his six sedentary obese men and on a program which involved an 1100 kcal expenditure per session, there was a loss of 5.9 kg of body fat and a gain of 0.2 kg of lean tissue. This was accompanied by a reduction in endogenous insulin requirement that has significant implication for individuals with glucose intolerance.

Questions concerning augmented appetite associated with increased energy expenditure are relevant, for many Americans wish to, or should, reduce body weight and, in particular, adiposity. Leon's report is not unique in demonstrating that habitually increased physical activity will result in weight loss, perhaps due to temporary appetite suppression. When a person recognizes a tendency for appetite reduction to occur after exercise, it may be helpful to schedule the activities prior to the meal in which overeating is most likely to occur.

Practical Applications

Many physicians, upon reviewing the preceding data, encourage their patients to engage in physical activities that can be included in already overcrowded life-styles. This is not easy, for the time, effort and resources involved are not inconsequential. Consideration must be given to the type, intensity, frequency and duration of activity as well as personal skills, preferences and available facilities.

Type and Intensity of Activities

In general, there is strong support for endurance-stimulating activities being more useful than those aimed at strength development, such as weight lifting. Use of the legs to carry body weight is advantageous, but rowing, paddling and swimming will give excellent general body conditioning with good cardiovascular training effects. Table 2 lists some, but by no means all, such vigorous activities with approximate kilocalorie per minute values ascribed to them.

Table 2. Types, Intensities and Energy Requirements of Some Recreational Activities

			Approx. kcal/min.
Most Demanding			
Cross Country Skiing	5	mph	11–12
Running	7	mph	12–14
Karate			10–13
Bicycling	13	mph	10–12
Basketball (full court)			10–12
Moderately Demanding			
Swimming (crawl, 50 meters/min)			9–11
Skating (vigorous)			9–10
Handball			9–11
Squash			10–12
Running/jogging	5.5 mph		10–12
Tennis (vigorous singles)			9–10
Downhill skiing with tight turns			8–10
Bicycling	11	mph	7–8
Racquetball			7–10
Less Demanding			
Walking	4.5 mph		6–7
Skating (moderately vigorous)			5–7
Tennis (moderately vigorous)			7–8
Canoeing	4	mph	7–8
Badminton (vigorous)			6–8
Folk (square) dancing			6–9

...ergy expenditure depends greatly upon the skill involved, eg, the ability to keep the ball in play in racquet sports. In proportion to the work rate involved, the effects of such useful activities as mowing the lawn, raking leaves, chopping wood, shoveling snow and turning over a compost pile can range from that of minor benefit to that which overtaxes the heart with narrowing of the coronary arteries. Before recommending high intensity activities, it is well to have a coronary risk estimation.[23] If the risk of developing coronary disease manifestations is above 8% to 12% in six years, on the basis of the Framingham Study tables,[23] a symptom- or sign-limited exercise tolerance test (treadmill or bicycle) is probably justified. This is particularly appropriate for a person who has been physically inactive, is obese, is under stress, highly competitive or a "Type A" personality,[7] or has a family history of CHD. The routine exercise testing of asymptomatic individuals at low risk for coronary disease detection alone does not appear to be cost-effective,[24] although it might serve as a strong stimulus for improving overall health and physical conditioning.

Duration and Frequency of Activities

Individual considerations influence the duration and frequency of physical activities. Racquet sports, which have considerable social as well as physiologic rewards, are usually scheduled for court time and may entail time spent in travel. Thus, the total duration for the activity is extended beyond a minimum, which may ultimately influence the frequency with which an individual can participate in the activity. Both a discrete warm-up and cool-down routine, varying from a few to 15 or more minutes, should be included in total time considerations, particularly before intense activities such as running or competitive sports.

The relative values of Frequency-Intensity-Duration and their interchangeability are not well-defined. To acquire the reduced coronary risk status implied by the studies of Morris[3,4] and Paffenbarger,[5] it is suggested that frequencies above twice a week and durations above 15 to 30 minutes are desirable at intensities requiring energy expenditures of 7 kcal/min or more. For higher intensities, the fitness benefits are acquired faster and may require fewer total expended calories. The number of overuse syndromes of musculo-skeletal origin, and even cardiovascular dysfunction or damage, increases with exercise of higher intensities especially, but also with the duration and even the frequency of the activity.

It is important to emphasize that patients should appreciate the long-term benefits to be acquired. Major increases in intensity, duration and frequency of physical activities should be staged gradually over a period of time. Thus, minor symptoms of intolerance can be recognized so that medical consultation and modification of the program, when indicated, will prevent significant discomfort, dysfunction or damage.

Programs for the Treatment of Coronary Heart Disease

Since World War II, the medical management of patients with acute coronary disease has been more aggressive. The goal has been to return the patient to a life-style that includes varying levels of physical activity, even including successful marathon running for a selected few. More recently, physical training has been added to the rehabilitation program for coronary bypass patients. Combined with those having an acute infarction, there are probably over a half million patients per year who may be candidates for a structured diet, exercise and life-style improvement program. Although some coronary patients will have severe limitations that make a formal exercise program a difficult and, at times, an unrewarding venture, there is considerable justification for low level reconditioning to enhance peripheral adaptation that will permit a more comfortable pursuit of the activities of daily living.

The mortality rate within cardiac rehabilitation programs with experienced staff has been declining and now appears to be less than one death incurred in well over 100,000 person-hours of supervised exercise programming.[25]

Table 3 illustrates a four phase progression of rehabilitation activities starting at the acute episode of myocardial infarction or bypass surgery. Such a division into phases is helpful chiefly for program planning because individualization should be paramount here, as in other areas of clinical management.

It is of utmost importance that the patient develops an understanding of the atherosclerotic process and its apparent basis in factors of life-style, rather than merely accepting it as an inexorable genetic predisposition with little capability for change. A rewarding exercise program, made as enjoyable as possible for each patient, can serve as the strongest means of support for correction of other risk factors such as diet, tobacco use, hypertension, adiposity and psychological stress. An attempt to reduce all risk factors simultaneously may be possible for some individuals; for many, however, it would be difficult to cope with more than diet and cessation of smoking, initially. Hopefully, this could be accomplished in a setting of reduced stress. Exercise is a "positive action that begets positive thoughts" for life-style modification.

For an in-patient, it must be recognized that the areas of infarction and surgical anastamoses need time to heal, so Phase I is aimed chiefly at avoiding deterioration, while activity must be limited. Passive and then active movements are used to maintain muscle strength and avoid later restrictions. An example is lateral, untilted head turning as an "Expressway Entry Exercise" to avoid later limitations. Deep breathing is important to avoid atelectasis and should be started before surgery, as an even earlier stage of programming.

After hospital discharge, it has been all too common to learn that a patient has become depressed and inactive, perhaps, in part, due to an overly solicitous family that tries to remove the patient from all possible stress. This may result in a sense of emasculation and/or loss of present and future control. The situation can often be avoided by having the "significant other" person present at the time of the "Low Level Exercise Tolerance Test (ETT)". The ETT demonstrates

Table 3. Four Phases of Cardiac Rehabilitation

	Entry Criteria	Education	Exercise	Exercise Tolerance Testing
Phase I "In-Hospital"	Myocardial Infarction (MI) Coronary Artery Bypass Surgery (CABG) Post Renal Transplant Hemodialysis	Individual and with "significant other" person Disease process Anatomy Pathophysiology Risk Factors Sex and the Heart Pulse taking Possibly in groups later	Passive ROM Active ROM Orthostatic Ambulation Stretching	Low Level, 3–6 METS (multiples of resting metabolic demands) prior to discharge or shortly thereafter to reassure patient, family and physician
Phase II "Continued Healing" until 8–12 weeks post MI, more rapid for post-CABG	Hospital Discharge Complete Phase I Sudden Death Survivor Severely Limited (Functional Aerobic Impairment of Dr. Bruce >35%) Uncontrolled hypertension (>240 systolic) Dysrhythmia Selected anginal syndromes Renal Dialysis, COPD	Individual and with "significant other" people Group classes Repeat and expand the above Diet and Stress Reinforcement	"Avoid deterioration" Low-level conditioning Abdominal Muscles started "Positive Actions Beget Positive Thoughts" to counteract depression	"Symptom Limited" to develop exercise prescription and evaluate other therapy at end of "healing phase"
Phase III "Training" or "Retraining"	Complete Phase II Stable Angina Post CABG "Medical Management" High CHD Risk or ischemic ETT	Group sessions including patient, family and friends Occasional individual and/or couple sessions	Symptom-Controlled or approximately 70–85% of achieved heart rate; adjusted to medications	"Symptom Limited" to "Max" every 3 to 12 months
Phase IV "Maintenance" or "Health Enhancement"	Complete Phase III As above plus those enjoying group setting	As above and with broader topic range	Symptom or Heart controlled or "released"	As above every 6 to 36 months as indicated

capabilities to pursue a modest program of home ambulation without adverse symptoms, blood pressure responses or electrocardiographic abnormalities of ischemia or dysrhythmia. Where transportation to a rehabilitation program is feasible, the further educational re-enforcement and monitored exercise can be a very positive element helping to counteract the almost universal depressive tendencies associated with a significant coronary disease diagnosis.

Along with occasional rehabilitation visits should go an expanded activity program during the "Continued Healing Phase" (II). Frequency of short slow walks can make up for intensity and duration, both of which will be expanded after healing is considered adequately secure.

The "Retraining Phase" (III) should usually be preceded by another evaluation of heart rate, blood pressure, symptoms and signs of adaptation or intolerance during another exercise tolerance test. This should be carried to an intensity level above that contemplated for the patient so that some "target" heart rate recommendations can be made ("maximum" or an advised "target range"). Over a period of months, some improvement should be realized. If no objective evidence of increased capability is found with reasonable patient compliance, it may be a strong indication that further studies will be helpful in determining optimal therapy. During the"Retraining Phase", a series of exercise stations, comprising a circuit of differing devices alternating the skeletal muscles used, can be an effective means of restoring total body conditioning. In the "Maintenance Phase" (IV), the emphasis shifts to those individual activities which continue to stimulate cardiovascular improvement, yet have the optimal pleasant elements of social interaction and appropriate game-type competition that will sustain lifelong involvement. The transition to these activities should be gradual and actively supported by the rehabilitation team so as to achieve the greatest benefit.

The objective of a structured program of diet education, life-style assessment and exercise therapy is to augment and support the individual patient's understanding and commitment to a change in life-style. Major assumption of responsibility for compliance by the patient and "significant other" people is necessary to achieve the long-term goals of risk reduction and health enhancement. Thus, efforts should be directed towards providing variety and enjoyment in both the diet and physical activities—the "smorgasbord approach". It was of great interest to find that Leren (personal communication, February 1976) had found in a previous trial, before the recent, more successful diet study,[2] that sustained cholesterol-lowering could be achieved by a program that permitted one "escape" meal of a less prudent type each week. The same approach appears important in the exercise regimen. Patients should not develop guilt as a result of an occasional break in an otherwise prescribed program of exercising at least every other day. This is particularly true when the patient becomes fatigued, over-extended, or impaired by any number of infections, and gastrointestinal or allergic disturbances. An exercise program that is reduced to walking, or near total avoidance of exertion, is sometimes indicated, particularly if it can result in a more prompt return to full activity. For the patient with established

...y disease, not amenable to or requiring bypass surgery (or balloon angioplasty), a more frequent exercise program of longer duration may be beneficial. The benefits may be equivalent to the morbidity and mortality reduction noted in the studies of Morris and Paffenbarger.[3-5]

The formulation of the activity prescription will be aided by exercise tolerance testing without or combined with radionuclide techniques. Although somewhat costly, these studies, when applied with thought, can serve as worthwhile stimuli for life-style change, as well as the basis for more exact and rational exercise and therapeutic prescriptions. It is important to recognize that exercise can be hazardous and deaths attributed to injudicious exercise are being reported.[26]

Needed Research

Although the Finnish[8] and Norwegian[2] studies show encouraging capabilities to alter the saturated fat in the diet, in a manner associated with a reduced incidence of heart attacks, they do not achieve a highly significant effect on overall mortality. Perhaps the Multiple Risk Factor Intervention Trial[27] soon to be reported, will provide more information on the dietary question. There are no large prospective intervention trials looking at the physical activity question known to be under way, although more data from the National Exercise and Heart Disease Project[12] and a World Health Organization Project may provide further data.

It would also be desirable to have more data on whether the exercising individual can tolerate, or "get away with", a diet less restricted in saturated fat and still avoid atherosclerotic and coronary disease manifestations.[28] As the scientific community plans for such additional research, it would seem prudent to assist patients in decreasing their tobacco use, hypertension, serum cholesterol (and probably their triglyceride) levels, and their body weight. An increase in habitual physical activity is also suggested not only for its potential to decrease coronary and other atherosclerotic disease, but to aid in the support of general mental and physical health and thus reduce expensive and depressing dependency.

Summary

A review of data from longitudinal studies and of intervention trials strongly suggest, but does not definitively prove, that an increase in habitual physical activity of an endurance-stimulating type is likely to reduce the risk of coronary heart disease and other atherosclerotic-thrombotic manifestations. Some mechanisms whereby this may take place have been proposed, but much more research is needed. The type, intensity, duration and frequency of exercises to be included in an activity program can vary according to individual interests and circumstances, but some general recommendations are becoming better defined. Above all, the activities should be of acceptable low hazard, rewarding and enjoyable.

Acknowledgement

Development of this review was supported in part by the Preventive Cardiology Academic Award, NHLBI, K-07-HL00660.

References

1. Hypertension Detection and Follow-Up Program Cooperative Group, NHLBI: Five-year findings of the Hypertension Detection and Follow-Up Program I & II. *JAMA* 242:2562-2577, 1979.
2. Hjermann I, Velve Byre K, Holme I, et al: Effect of diet and smoking intervention on the incidence of coronary heart disease. *Lancet* 8259:1303-1310, 1981.
3. Morris JN, Chave SPW, Adam C, et al: Vigorous exercise in leisure-time and the incidence of coronary heart-disease. *Lancet* 7799:333-339, 1973.
4. Morris JN, Everitt MG, Pollard R, et al: Vigorous exercise in leisure-time: Protection against coronary heart disease. *Lancet* 8206:1207-1210, 1980.
5. Paffenbarger RS, Wing AL, Hyde RT: Physical activity as an index of heart attack risk in college alumni. *Am J Epidemiol* 108:161-175, 1978.
6. Kannel WB, Sorlie MS: Some health benefits of physical activity-The Framingham study. *Arch Intern Med* 139:857-861, 1979.
7. Rosenman RH, The influence of different exercise patterns on the incidence of coronary heart disease in the Western Collaborative Group Study, in Brunner D, Jokl E (eds): *Physical Activity and Aging*. Baltimore, University Park Press, 1970, pp 267-273.
8. Kallio V, Hamalainen H, Hakkila J, et al: Reduction in sudden death by a multifactional intervention programme after acute myocardial infarction. *Lancet* 2:1091-1097, 1979.
9. Kentala E: Physical fitness and feasibility of physical rehabilitation after myocardial infarction in men of working age. *Ann Clin Res* 4 (suppl 9): 1-84, 1972.
10. Rechnitzer PA, Sangal SA, Cunningham DA, et al: A controlled prospective study of the effect of endurance training on the recurrence rate of myocardial infarction. *Am J Epidemiol* 102:358-365, 1975.
11. Wilhelmsen L, Sanne H, Elmfeldt D, et al: A controlled trial of physical training after myocardial infarction. *Prev Med* 4:491-508, 1975.
12. Shaw LW: The National Exercise and Heart Disease Project: Effect of a prescribed supervised exercise program on mortality and cardiovascular morbidity in patients after a myocardial infarction. *Am J Cardiol* 48:39-46, 1981.
13. Fox SM, Naughton JP, Gorman PA: Physical activity and cardiovascular health. *Mod Concepts Cardiovasc Dis* 41:17-30, 1972.
14. Shephard RJ: *Ischemic Heart Disease and Exercise*. Chicago, Year Book Med Publ, 1981, p. 428.
15. Kramsch DM, Aspen AJ, Abramowitz BM, et al: Reduction of coronary atherosclerosis by moderate conditioning exercise in monkeys on an atherogenic diet. *N Engl J Med* 305:1483-1489, 1981.
16. Selvester R, Camp J, Sanmarco M: Effects of exercise training on progression of documented coronary arteriosclerosis in men. *Ann NY Acad Sci* 301:495-508, 1977.
17. Ehsani AA, Heath GW, Hagberg JM, et al: Effects of 12 months of intense exercise training on ischemic ST-segment depression in patients with coronary artery disease. *Circulation* 64:1116-1124, 1981.
18. Haskell WL: Influence of habitual physical activity on blood lipids and lipoproteins, in Cohen LS, Mock MB, Ringqvist I (eds): *Physical Conditioning and Cardiovascular Rehabilitation*, New York, John Wiley, 1981, pp. 87-102.
19. Miller GJ, Miller NE: Plasma high density lipoprotein concentrations and development of ischemic heart disease. *Lancet* 1:16-19, 1975.
20. Carew TE, Koschinsky T, Hayes SB, et al: A mechanism by which high density lipoproteins may slow the atherogenic process. *Lancet* 1:1315-1317, 1976.

21. Leon AS, Conrad J. Hunninglake DB, et al: Effects of a vigorous walking program on body composition and carbohydrate and lipid metabolism of obese young men. *Am J Clin Nutr* 32:1779–1787, 1979.

22. Allison TG, Iammarino RM, Metz KF, et al: Failure of exercise to increase high density lipoprotein cholesterol. *J Card Rehab* 1:257–265, 1981.

23. American Heart Association: *Coronary Risk Handbook: Estimating Risk of Coronary Heart Disease in Daily Practice*, Dallas, Texas, 1973, p.35.

24. Bruce RA, DeRouen TA, Hossack KF: Value of maximal exercise tests in risk assessment of primary coronary heart disease events in healthy men: Five Years experience of the Seattle Heart Watch Study. *Amer J Card* 46:371–378, 1980.

25. Haskell WL: Cardiovascular complications during exercise training of cardiac patients. *Circulation* 57:920–925, 1978.

26. Thompson PD, Funk EJ, Carleton RA, et al: Incidence of death during jogging in Rhode Island from 1975 through 1980. *JAMA* 247:2535–2538,1982.

27. Forum: The Multiple Risk Factor Intervention Trial (MRFIT). The methods and impact over four years. *Prev Med* 10:387–553, 1981.

28. Wood PD, Haskell WL: Interrelation of physical activity and nutrition on lipid metabolism, in White PLW, Mondeika TM (eds): *Diet and Exercise: Synergism in Health Maintenance*. Chicago, American Medical Association, 1982, pp 39–47.

EXERCISE AND DIET IN THE THERAPY OF DIABETES*

Neil B. Ruderman, MD, DPhil,** Stephen H. Schneider, MD,***
Louis Amoroso, MD*** and Dieter Kramsch, MD**

Introduction

The increasing evidence that microvascular disease and perhaps other long-term complications of diabetes are related to the degree of hyperglycemia has resulted in an intense effort to improve metabolic control in the diabetic.[1] Thus, home monitoring programs and insulin infusion pumps have been developed and an increasing percentage of Type I (insulin-dependent) diabetics are presently treated with multiple-dose insulin regimens. At the same time, there has been a renewed interest in the use of diet and exercise in diabetic therapy. The basic recommendations for the diabetic diet have been somewhat modified and the differing dietary needs of insulin-dependent and non-insulin dependent (Type II) diabetics have been clarified. (In the previously-used terminology, Type I and Type II diabetes were referred to as "juvenile-onset" and "maturity-onset", respectively.[2]) In addition, a number of investigators have begun to evaluate the potential of regular exercise for both improving glucose homeostasis and preventing or retarding the development of atherosclerotic vascular disease and its complications.

The principal objective of this review is to examine the present status of diet and exercise in the therapy of diabetes. Newer developments and concepts will be stressed and some of the key issues which remain to be explored will be indicated. As several excellent and comprehensive reviews on diet therapy have recently appeared,[3-7] and as the principal interest of the authors is in the use of exercise, its role will be evaluated somewhat more extensively.

Diet

Insulin-dependent Diabetes (Type I)
The principal objectives of diet therapy in the insulin-dependent diabetic are (1) to maintain body weight and/or growth and (2) to tailor calorie intake to the patient's insulin regimen and life style so as to achieve optimal glycemic control. To attain these goals, the patient has to carefully balance his food intake and insulin regimen. Thus, insulin and/or diet often have to be adjusted as a

---

*The paper was presented by Dr. Ruderman.
**Boston University Medical Center, Boston, Massachusetts
***New Jersey College of Medicine, Piscataway, New Jersey

consequence or in anticipation of such events as exercise, illness and delayed meals. The specifics of how a patient accomplishes this are discussed elsewhere.[3-7] Suffice it to say that with the increasing use of home blood glucose monitoring and multidose insulin regimens and insulin infusion pumps, it has become possible to achieve far tighter control with more flexibility in diet than has heretofore been possible.

The composition of the diet recommended for both Type I and Type II diabetics has changed significantly in the past ten years. The classic recommendation that dietary carbohydrate must be restricted in order to diminish hyperglycemia has been rejected; indeed, it has been pointed out that the high fat diets necessitated by such carbohydrate restriction are likely to be atherogenic.[3] A comparison of typical diabetic diets currently used with diets prescribed 15 years ago is presented in Table 1. In addition to the shift in percent of dietary fat and carbohydrate, it is now recommended that at least 50% of the fat ingested be in the form of unsaturated fatty acids; also, the ingestion of alcoholic beverages in prescribed amounts, with the approval of the physician, is permitted.

Table 1. Recommended Composition of the Typical Diabetic Diet

	Traditional	New
	Percent of Total Calories	
Carbohydrate	35–40	45–55
Fat	40–45	25–35
Protein	16–21	12–24
Alcohol	0	0–6
	Ratio	
Fat (Unsaturated/Total)	Not specified	0.5–0.7

Adapted from West.[3] The increase in carbohydrate in the present-day diet is totally in its component of starch and other polysaccharides. An even higher percentage of carbohydrate and a lower percentage as fat would probably be desirable, however, such a diet would seldom be possible in Western society because of traditional eating habits.

Non-insulin-dependent Diabetes (Type II)

Type II diabetics are typically over 40 years of age and somewhat obese. Unlike the Type I patient, they are not totally or near-totally deficient in insulin; in fact, circulating insulin levels may be high. The central problem in many of these individuals appears to be insulin resistance, secondary to obesity and/or the prolonged ingestion of excess calories.[3-8] A similar pattern of insulin resistance is seen in non-diabetics who are obese; however, plasma insulin levels in these individuals are sufficiently high to maintain normoglycemia. Plasma insulin in the obese diabetic is generally somewhat lower than in his non-obese counterpart; nevertheless, it may still be markedly increased in comparison to levels in a non-obese, normoglycemic individual of the same age.

The objective of diet therapy in the Type II diabetic is to diminish insulin resistance so that endogenous insulin can maintain glucose homeostasis. Thus, if the patient is obese,[3-7] or sometimes even normal weight,[8] reduced calorie intake is prescribed. In contrast to the Type I diabetic, the precise timing and composition of meals, day-to-day consistency of calorie intake and adjustments for exercise are not crucial for the Type II diabetic, provided the patient is not receiving insulin. As pointed out by Davidson,[9] and as illustrated in Table 2, weight reduction regimens may allow obese diabetics treated with insulin to be treated with diet alone. Characteristically, these patients achieve better glycemic control with weight loss than with insulin therapy. In addition, the weight loss may cause a dramatic improvement in various risk factors for cardiovascular disease including hypertension and hypertriglyceridemia. Interestingly, many of these improvements occur within one to two weeks and are maintained even though ideal weight has not been achieved. The long-term outcome in individuals who continue on these diets and/or maintain their weight loss is not known.

Other dietary approaches presently under investigation in the diabetic include high fiber diets[10] and the use of an orally administered intestinal glucosidase inhibitor (Acarbose). The latter, like the high fiber diet, retards glucose absorption from the gut and diminishes hyperglycemia following meals. The question has also been raised as to whether the composition of the western diet, and particularly its sucrose content, has contributed to the apparently increasing incidence of diabetes.[11] Although the epidemiological evidence supporting such a hypothesis is equivocal,[11] it is noteworthy that some individuals developed marked hyperinsulinemia when on diets containing even normal amounts of sucrose.[12] Whether these individuals are more likely to develop diabetes if they continue to ingest sucrose is not known.

Table 2. Effect of Strict Diet Therapy on an Obese Patient with Type II Diabetes

Date	Wt. lbs	Insulin U/day	BP	Fasting Glucose mb/dl	HbA$_1$
1/79	203	25	130/95	277	10.9
11/79	198	44	140/85	196	10.1
4/80	188	0	118/70	140	5.4
6/80	181	0	120/77	120	7.6
9/80	183	0	114/70	139	7.2
3/81	194	0	160/90	128	8.4
7/81	192	0		218	9.8

The patient, a 58 year old diabetic of 4 years duration, was taken off insulin in the hospital and placed on a 400-calorie, high-protein diet. Improvement in glycemic status was evident within one week. When she regained weight both her hyperglycemia and hypertension returned.

Exercise

Glucose Homeostasis

Physical training increases insulin sensitivity in normal man[13,14] and for this reason its effect on glucose homeostasis has been assessed in patients with Type II diabetes. The results have been equivocal. In a small group of previously sedentary Type II diabetic men, only a modest improvement in glucose tolerance was observed,[15] whereas in an equally small group of obese diabetics, no improvement was observed.[16] In contrast, a near normalization of glucose tolerance has been reported in a large group of middle-aged men with chemical diabetes.[17] Whether selected Type II diabetics will show a more marked improvement with physical training or whether improved glucose homeostasis can be more readily demonstrated using indices other than the glucose tolerance test remain to be determined. An examination of the latter possibility may be especially critical since, in the studies reported to date, glucose tolerance has only been assessed several days after the last bout of exercise; therefore, acute benefits derived from regular exercise could have been missed (see below).

Cardiovascular Disease

A potentially important role of regular exercise in the diabetic is in the prevention or retardation of cardiovascular disease and its complications. Nearly 70% of all diabetics die of some form of cardiovascular disease. The principal cause is atherosclerosis, which morphologically is very similar to that seen in non-diabetics.[18] As shown in the Framingham study,[19] the relative incidence of atherosclerotic cerebrovascular, peripheral vascular and coronary artery disease is more than twice as great in diabetics 45–74 years of age as in the general population, and this is irrespective of whether the patient is treated with diet, oral agents or insulin.

The purpose of this section is to examine the limited evidence that chronic endurance exercise might protect the diabetic against atherosclerotic vascular disease. For the most part, the studies which will be reviewed have been carried out in normal subjects; however, there is little reason to believe the findings would not also apply to the diabetic.

Epidemiological Studies. Nearly 15 years ago, Morris et al[20] pointed out that the mortality rate of sedentary London bus drivers was substantially higher than that of more active conductors. Although later studies have generally supported the notion that physically-active people are less likely to die prematurely of cardiovascular disease, it is still unclear whether this is due to an effect of physical training or whether physically-active individuals somehow differ from their sedentary counterparts.[21] To a great extent, this problem was overcome in an ongoing study of Harvard College graduates, in which prior family history and athletic capability were considered. As reported by Paffenbarger et al,[22] the incidence of first heart attacks was significantly less in more active individuals and maximum benefit was observed in subjects who exercised the equivalent of 2,000 kcal/week or more. The beneficial effects of exercise were seen in cigarette smokers, hypertensives and diabetics. The number of diabetics studied was small, however, and no attempt was made to determine if the less active diabetics had vascular complications which prevented them from exercise (R. Paffenbarger, MD, written communication, April 1980).

Coronary Risk Factors. Epidemiological studies have delineated a number of abnormalities which single out the patient at risk for coronary artery and other forms of cardiovascular disease. Each of these "risk factors" is independently associated with an increased likelihood of cardiovascular mortality and/or morbidity. Of the factors studied, hypertriglyceridemia, diminished HDL cholesterol, hypertension, obesity and possibly an increase in plasma cholesterol and inactivity are more common in the diabetic.[1,15,17-19]* The potential benefit of endurance exercise stems from the fact that it favorably alters all or nearly all of these risk factors in the general population.[15,23,24] Studies in diabetics are limited; however, the findings of a single investigation carried out in five middle-aged patients with Type II diabetes suggest that the effect of training on plasma triglycerides, and possibly cholesterol, is identical to that observed in the non-diabetic.[15]

Recent investigations[25] have also called attention to the role of platelets and the endothelial cell in the pathogenesis of atherosclerosis and have stimulated an intense interest in abnormalities of hemostasis. The diabetic is particularly noteworthy because of abnormalities in the function and metabolism of both the platelet and the endothelial cell, including diminished thromboxane production, a decreased ability to form prostacyclin, an increase in Von Willibrand's factor, and a decrease in fibrinolytic activity in blood.[26] The effect of endurance exercise on these parameters has received little attention, although recently it has been shown that training increases the fibrinolytic response in normal man following venous occlusion.[27] In addition, we have found that training causes an increase in fibrinolytic activity, as assessed by euglobulin lysis time, in patients with Type II diabetes (unpublished data, September 1981).

Animal Studies. Although investigations in man have provided circumstantial evidence that endurance exercise protects against cardiovascular disease, further studies in man are unlikely to produce direct proof of such a protective effect; nor are they likely to explain its mechanism. For this reason, the effect of endurance exercise has been recently studied in experimental animals. A protective effect of training on myocardial infarct size in young animals following an experimental coronary occlusion has been described.[28,29] Additionally, train-

---

*Note: Most epidemiological studies have evaluated Type II diabetics. Different factors may play a more critical role in the Type I diabetic, who is also more predisposed to cardiovascular disease.

ing has been shown to increase the activity of aortic acid cholesterol esterase.[30] This enzyme is thought to play a key role in cellular cholesterol disposition and is depressed in diabetic rats.[31]

Particularly relevant to this discussion are the studies of Kramsch et al[32] in which the effect of physical training on the development of atherosclerosis was examined in the Macaca fascicularis monkey. Monkeys were placed on atherogenic diets which had previously been shown to produce severe atherosclerosis within 18 months. One group was maintained in its usual state (sedentary) and the other was made to run on a specially constructed treadmill three times per week for at least 30 minutes. When they were sacrificed after 1½ years, the exercised monkeys had a slower pulse rate, indicating they were physically conditioned. In addition, the severity of coronary and peripheral atherosclerosis as judged by gross appearance, light microscopy and the biochemical composition of various arteries was much less than in the sedentary group (Table 3). Total plasma cholesterol ($\sim$ 600 mg/dl) and LDL cholesterol were similar in the two groups, suggesting that differences in some other factor(s) was responsible. Diabetic monkeys develop more severe vascular diseases than comparable controls when placed on an atherogenic diet.[33,34] Whether physical training would provide any protective effect remains to be determined.

Table 3. Collagen Content of Various Arteries: Effect of Exercise in Monkeys on an Atherogenic Diet

	Collagen (μg/cm length/kg body weight) Atherogenic Diet	
	Sedentary	Exercised
Thoracic aorta	782	376*
Abdominal aorta	963	441*
Carotid	151	76*

Data are those of Kramsch, Aspen, Abramowitz, Abel and Hood (unpublished) and are for 6–10 monkeys. See text for details.
*$p < 0.05$ is sedentary group.

Physical Training in Diabetic Man

The Piscataway Study
Endurance physical activities such as running, swimming and cycling increase an individual's capacity for aerobic exercise and cause multiple adaptations in the cardiovascular system. In addition, they produce enzymatic alterations in skeletal muscle which increase its ability to carry out oxidative metabolism. The few studies carried out in diabetics suggest that their response to such an exercise regimen is qualitatively similar to that of non-diabetics.[35] In order to assess the effect of such exercise on a number of coronary risk factors and hemostatic parameters, we initiated a physical training program for Type II

Table 4. Characteristics of Control and Diabetic Patients Before and After Six weeks of Training

	Control (n=10)		Diabetic (n=16)	
	Pre	Post	Pre	Post
Age (years)	46			
Wt (kg)	80.5	80.6	78.8	79.3
VO_2 max (ml/kg/min)	33	37†	25*	30†
Heart rate at VO_2 max	181	182	162*	160
Fasting plasma glucose (mg/dl)	99	92	191*	178†
Hemoglobin Ac_1 (%)	7.5	7.6	12.2*	10.7†

Patients performed aerobic exercise at 60–70% VO_2 max for 45 minutes, three times a week. See text for details.
* $p < 0.05$ vs control
† $p < 0.05$ vs pre-training value

diabetics which is presently operative at New Jersey College of Medicine in Piscataway. The characteristics of the first 10 control and 16 diabetic patients to complete six weeks of training are noted in Table 4. As in previous studies,[15,17] the diabetics achieved a significant improvement in maximum aerobic capacity. Approximately one-third of them showed some improvement in glucose tolerance and fasting plasma glucose (both determined four days after the last bout of exercise). For the group as a whole, the improvement in glucose tolerance was not significant; however, the decrease in fasting plasma glucose was small. On the other hand, the percent of glycosylated hemoglobin was significantly decreased in the diabetics after training, suggesting that their average plasma glucose concentration during the previous 4 to 6 weeks had been lowered. If this notion is correct; it would indicate that the improvement in glycemic status is due to a relatively transient effect of exercise, that it is independent of the degree of training achieved, and that it may be missed if glucose tolerance testing is performed several days after the last bout of exercise. Further evidence is needed to corroborate this, however. Preliminary data also indicate that the training regimen used here causes a substantial decrease in plasma triglycerides but that it has little, if any, effect on either total plasma cholesterol or cholesterol in the HDL fraction.

Of especial interest was the finding that, as a group, the Type II diabetics had a lower aerobic work capacity (VO_2 max) than the controls even though they were closely matched for age, weight, and physical activity history. A similar observation has been made in chemical diabetics by Saltin et al.[17] The cause of this decrease in aerobic capacity is unclear. Heart rate (Table 4), minute volume and plasma lactate (data not shown) were all lower in the diabetics during maximal exercise; however, it remains to be determined whether these changes were the cause or the result of the diminished aerobic capacity. None of the patients had clinically evident autonomic neuropathy and only 25% of them had a diminished R-R interval variation with respiration.

Practical Considerations

Special precautions should be taken in previously sedentary diabetics about to embark on an exercise program. Because of the high incidence of chronically silent cardiovascular disease, we believe stress-testing should be carried out in all patients over the age of 40 as well as in younger diabetics with other coronary risk factors. Exercise sessions should probably be omitted in very hot weather due to the greater risk of postural hypotension, and during intermittent illnesses when the risk of poor control and dehydration is high. At the very least, warm-up and warm-down sessions of five minutes or more should be part of the patient's regimen. Diabetics with significant sensory neuropathy should avoid jogging and other exercises which could severely traumatize the feet. Likewise, intensive exercise should be discouraged in the presence of proliferative retinopathy due to the risk of hemorrhage. Additional precautions must be taken in patients treated with insulin, as they may develop hypoglycemia both during or following exercise. Such individuals should always have available a ready source of carbohydrate as well as diabetic identification. In addition, if hypoglycemia is a recurrent problem, they must be taught to ingest carbohydrate or to diminish their insulin dose prior to exercise. Chemstrips or some other home-monitoring system may be particularly useful in assessing whether vague symptoms are due to hypoglycemia.

In our opinion, exercise should be performed at least three times per week if a training effect is desired and its duration and intensity should be individualized for each patient. We have found that the standard heart rate tables are not useful for judging the intensity of exercise in a diabetic. A simple formula which has worked well for us and which both correlates with exercise at approximately 70% of maximum aerobic capacity and causes a modest increase in systolic pressure is as follows:

$$\text{Target heart rate} = \text{Basal pulse rate} + 0.75 (\text{Maximum} - \text{Basal pulse rate})$$

Summary

The role of diet and exercise in the therapy of diabetes has been reviewed. Particular attention was focused on its potential role in improving glycemic status and diminishing the risk of atherosclerotic cardiovascular disease in the Type II diabetic. Ongoing work aimed at assessing the effect of exercise on coronary risk factors and glucose homeostasis should help to determine its utility and establish what special precautions are needed in this patient population. Initial studies suggest the Type II diabetic has a lower maximum aerobic capacity than an age and weight matched control. The reason for this remains to be determined.

Acknowledgment

Supported in part by USPHS grants AM 19514, AM 26894 and HL 18381.

References

1. Brownlee M, Cerami A: The biochemistry of the complications of diabetes. *Ann Rev Biochem* 50:385–432, 1981.
2. National Diabetes Data Group: Classification and diagnosis of diabetes and other classes of glucose intolerance. *Diabetes* 28:1039–1057, 1979.
3. West KM: Recent trends in dietary management, in Podolsky S, (ed): *Clinical Diabetes: Modern Management*. New York, Appleton-Century-Crofts, 1980, pp 67–81.
4. Davidson MD: *Diabetes Mellitus: Diagnosis and Treatment*. New York, John Wiley and Sons, 1981, vol 1, pp 48–108.
5. Hadden DR, Wilson EA: Dietary management of diabetes mellitus. *Proc Nutr Soc* 40:247–255, 1981.
6. Arky RA: Current principles of dietary therapy of diabetes mellitus. *Med Clin North Am* 62:655–662, 1978.
7. Skyler JS: Nutritional management of diabetes, in Katzen HM, Mahler RJ, (eds): *Diabetes, Obesity and Vascular Disease*. New York, John Wiley and Sons, 1978, pp 645–698.
8. Ruderman NB, Schneider SH, Berchtold P: The metabolically-obese, normal-weight individual. *Am J Clin Nutr* 34:1617–1621, 1981.
9. Davidson, JK: Controlling diabetes with diet therapy. *Postgrad Med* 59:114–122, 1976.
10. Anderson JW, Ward K: Long term effects of high-carbohydrate, high-fiber diets on glucose and lipid metabolism. *Diabetes Care* 1:293, 1978.
11. Baird JD: Diet and the development of clinical diabetes in man. *Proc Nutr Soc* 40:213–217, 1981.
12. Reiser S, Handler HB, Gardner LB, et al: Isocaloric exchange of dietary sucrose and starch in humans. II. Effect on fasting blood insulin, glucose and glucagon and glucose response to a sucrose load. *Am J Clin Nutr* 32:2206–2216, 1979.
13. Lohmann D, Liebold F, Heilmann W, et al: Diminished insulin response in highly trained athletes. *Metabolism* 27:521–524, 1978.
14. Bjorntorp P: The effects of exercise on plasma insulin. *Int J Sports Med* 2:125–129, 1981.
15. Ruderman NB, Ganda OP, Johansen K: The effect of physical training on glucose tolerance and plasma lipids in maturity-onset diabetes. *Diabetes* 23 (suppl 1):89–92, 1979.
16. Bjorntorp P, Dejounge K, Sjöström L, et al: Physical training in human obesity. II. Effects on plasma insulin in glucose intolerant subjects without hyperinsulinemia. *Scand J Clin Lab Invest* 32:41–45, 1973.
17. Saltin B, Lindgarde F, Houston M, et al: Physical training and glucose tolerance in middle-aged men with chemical diabetes. *Diabetes* (suppl 1): 30–32, 1979.
18. Jarrett RJ, Keen H: Diabetes and atherosclerosis, in Keen H, Jarrett J (eds): *Complications of Diabetes*. London, Arnold, 1975, pp 179–203.
19. Kannel WB, McGee DL: Diabetes and cardiovascular disease. The Framingham study. *JAMA* 241:2035–2038, 1979.
20. Morris JM, Kagan A, Pattison DC, et al: Incidence and prediction of ischemic heart disease in London busmen. *Lancet* 2:553–559, 1966.
21. Froelicher VF: Exercise and the prevention of coronary atherosclerotic heart disease. *Cardiovasc Clin* 9:3, 13–23, 1978.
22. Paffenbarger RS, Wing AL, Hyde RT: Physical activity as an index of heart attack risk in college alumni. *Am J Epidemiol* 108:161–175, 1978.

23. Wood PD, Haskell W, Klein H, et al: The distribution of plasma lipoproteins in middle-aged male runners. *Metabolism* 25:1249–1257, 1976.

24. Lopez-SA, Vial R, Balart L, et al: Effect of exercise and physical fitness on serum lipids and lipoproteins. *Atherosclerosis* 20:1–9, 1974.

25. Ross R: The arterial wall and atherosclerosis. *Ann Rev Med* 30:1–15, 1979.

26. Colwell JA, Halushka PJ: Platelet function in diabetes mellitus. *Brit J Haematol* 44:521–526, 1980.

27. Williams RS, Logue EE, Lewis JL, et al: Physical conditioning augments the fibrinolytic response to venous occlusion in healthy adults, *N Engl J Med* 302:987–991, 1980.

28. Scheuer J, Tipton CM: Cardiovascular adaptations to physical training. *Ann Rev Physiol* 39:221–251, 1977.

20. McElroy CL, Gissen SA, Fishbein MC: Exercise-induced reduction in myocardial infarct size after coronary occlusion in the rat. *Circulation* 57:958–962, 1978.

30. Wolinsky H, Goldfischer S, Katz D, et al: Effects of regular physical activity in hydrolase activities of the rat aorta. *Circulation* (suppl 21):167, 1979.

31. Wolinsky H, Goldfischer S, Capron L, et al: Hydrolase activities in the rat aorta. I. Effect of diabetes mellitus and insulin treatment. *Circ Res* 42:821–831, 1978.

32. Kramsch DM, Aspen AJ, Abramowitz BM, et al: Prevention of stenosing atherosclerotic disease of the coronary artery by moderate conditioning exercise in nonhuman primates in atherogenic duct. *N Engl J Med* 305:1483–1489, 1981.

33. Lehner NDM, Clarkson TB, Lofland HB: The effect of insulin deficiency, hypothyroidism and hypertension in atherosclerosis in the squirrel monkey. *Exp Molec Pathol* 15:230–244, 1971.

34. Lehner NDM: Effect of alloxan diabetes on atherosclerosis in squirrel monkeys. *Fed Proc* 34:876, 1975.

35. Richter EA, Ruderman NB, Schneider SH: Diabetes and exercise. *Am J Med* 70:201–208, 1981.

THE ROLE OF DIET AND ACTIVITY IN THE TREATMENT OF OSTEOPOROSIS

Robert P. Heaney, MD*

Introduction

Definition. It is important to establish at the outset that osteoporosis is not a specific disease but an end-state of the skeleton, in which the amount of structural bony material has been reduced to the point where fractures occur with relatively minor trauma. There are probably several osteoporotic syndromes, and undoubtedly many etiologies. They all have in common the fact that, while skeletal mass may be adequate for routine, everyday activity, it is no longer sufficient to withstand the infrequent strains of falls or other minor injuries.

The most common form of osteoporosis is that which occurs in postmenopausal women and, to a lesser extent and at a later age, in elderly men as well. Both sexes lose bone from about age 35 onwards, but the postmenopausal acceleration of bone loss in women is substantial (on the order of 2% per year immediately following estrogen deprivation); hence bone mass is reduced to a far greater extent in women than in men of corresponding age.

Distinction Between Prevention and Treatment. The term "treatment" often includes notions of both prevention and remediation. The goal of prevention is the maintenance of peak adult bone mass, or at least the slowing of age-related loss. This topic has been discussed by Whedon in an earlier chapter.[1] The topic which I will address is the treatment of the established disease, ie, treatment of the patient who already has bone mass reduced to the point where one or more fractures have occurred and disability has resulted. The goals of such remedial treatment fall into five discrete categories:

1) symptomatic treatment of the acute fracture and of chronic disability;
2) rehabilitation after fracture or as compensation for deformity;
3) arrest of further bone loss;
4) restoration of lost bone mass; and
5) restoration of damaged skeletal architecture.

It is probably apparent that no remedy can produce all of these effects. Although it may be less obvious, it is important to stress that for some of those goals, no effective treatment is available at all. Further, it is necessary to add that what may work as prevention, may well not work as remedy.

Status of Current Knowledge. There have been very few studies of the effect of either diet or exercise in the treatment of established osteoporosis in elderly

---

*Creighton University, Omaha, Nebraska

persons; hence, there is very little factual information available. Data obtained from studies on mechanisms of bone loss or on the physiology of bone remodeling may be of value in the discussion of treatment of individuals with osteoporosis.

There are several reasons for this unsatisfactory state of knowledge. Osteoporosis is not a very glamorous disorder, and although afflicting many millions of individuals and costing the U.S. well in excess of one billion dollars per year in direct costs alone, it has not captured much popular attention. Further, it is a slowly progressive disorder, and, if it responds to treatment at all, the response tends to be equally as slow, so that studies are difficult to perform, inordinately time consuming, and correspondingly expensive. Additionally, it has only been within the past ten years that it is possible to measure bone mass with enough precision to allow the detection of changes produced by various forms of treatment. Finally, until very recently, bone physiology was so poorly understood that there was a tendency to misinterpret the findings obtained from newly developed, more sensitive methods.

This last point is worth further elaboration because it explains some of the misinformation which exists in our textbooks and even in the more recent literature. Bone undergoes continuous remodeling, as do most body tissues. The amount of mineralized bone at any time is influenced both by the rate of remodeling (which determines how much bone can be measured), and by the balance between the destructive and reparative components of remodeling (which determines real changes in bone mass). Until recently, we had failed adequately to recognize the significance of the former component, and had attributed all measured changes in bone mass to a (presumed) change in bone remodeling balance favoring either formation (repair) or resorption (destruction). It turns out that this was not always the case.

The problem can be best illustrated by analogy with a hotel in which a certain fraction of the rooms are always being remodeled or redecorated. If there are 500 guest rooms in the hotel, and 10% are out of service at any one time because of remodeling, then the management has effectively only 450 rooms available for use. If the remodeling rate is reduced from 10% to 5% at any one time, the management will appear to have gained 25 rooms, or an increase of slightly more than 5%, and if remodeling were to stop altogether for a time, there would be an apparent increase of a full 50 rooms. But of course, there really isn't any more hotel space; and the actual number of rooms remains unchanged. (Further, there are additional consequences of not keeping the rooms attractive and in good repair.)

Many influences, including diet and exercise, alter the rate of bone remodeling, without necessarily altering the remodeling balance. As the amount of bone being remodeled changes, there will be a change in the amount of resting bone, *but not in the sum total of resting and remodeling bone.* With modern, sensitive methods, it is now possible to detect these changes. The observed change often represents only a shift to a new steady state and not a continuing favorable imbalance as believed previously. Such an effect is now referred to as a "remodeling transient", or "filling up the remodeling space."[2]

Role of Diet and Exercise in Development of Osteoporosis

Status of Current Knowledge. The reasons for the universal loss in bone mass after age 35 are not known with certainty. It is probable, in both sexes, that the principal underlying reason is a decline in physical activity. Superimposed on that underlying, exercise-related factor in women is the loss of estrogen at menopause. This loss results in an immediate deterioration of calcium balance performance, ie, the woman absorbs calcium less efficiently from her diet, and excretes it more readily through the kidney. The combined result of these two changes is that the effective dietary requirement for calcium increases substantially in the absence of estrogen.[3] The median calcium intake for postmenopausal women in the U.S. (500 mg) is well below the current Recommended Dietary Allowance (800 mg), and is probably only about one-third of what it ought to be in order to offset this estrogen-related deterioration in calcium utilization (1,500 mg). Thus, age-related bone loss in North America is probably a composite of reduced mechanical stress and inadequate calcium intake, the latter factor aggravated by menopausal loss of estrogens in women.

Bone remodeling rate is important in this context because it determines how fast bone mass will change in response to declining activity. With reduced physical activity, the average packet of remodeling within the skeleton restores less bone in the formative phase than was removed in the prior resorptive phase. Thus, every time a unit of bone remodels in an aging person, some bone is lost. Consequently, as the rate of remodeling increases, bone loss also increases; conversely, as the rate of remodeling decreases, decline of bone mass also diminishes.

How do diet and exercise interact in this situation? Whedon has explored this relationship,[1] so suffice it to say here that there is always some phase lag between the amount of bone we actually have and the amount we actually need for everyday use, ie, it takes a finite period of time for the body to alter skeletal mass, either upwards or downwards, in response to changing mechanical utilization. With aging, daily mechanical stresses decline, slowly but progressively, and skeletal mass declines in parallel. With a nominally *adequate* dietary intake, the phase lag between decline in mechanical stresses and in skeletal mass will be of a certain duration. Available evidence does not permit fixing this duration with certainty, but it could easily be as much as 9–12 months. That means simply that at any given time, an aging person has the amount of skeleton which would have been necessary 9–12 months earlier. In terms of skeletal mass, this is equivalent to as much as 2% to 5% of the total mass. If the dietary calcium intake is *inadequate*, then remodeling is speeded up, and the phase lag is shortened; conversely, if there is a *surplus* of calcium in the diet and remodeling is suppressed, then the phase lag is lengthened.

Although dietary factors may not be able to prevent age-related bone loss, they appear to be important in determining how rapidly the decline in skeletal mass follows the decline in physical activity with age. Calcium intakes ranging from high to low could be responsible for as much as a 5% to 10% difference in skeletal mass at any given age. Differences of this magnitude may well be crucial in terms of fracture susceptibility.

Role of Diet and Exercise in Remedial Treatment of Osteoporosis

Exercise. Potential bone mass within genotypic limits is related to three factors: mechanical load, availability of raw materials, and rate of bone remodeling. As indicated earlier, mechanical stress is probably the most important determinant of skeletal mass, other factors being equal. Ideally, treatment for osteoporosis should include a significant increase in mechanical loading of the skeleton. However, this is often not practicable, both because of lifelong sedentary habits of the patients, and because of the pain and disability caused by osteoporosis-related fractures. Studies have been conducted which show an apparent increase in total body bone mass as a result of exercise,[4] and it is reasonable to expect such a finding. It is not certain, however, whether the results represent anything more than a remodeling transient or, if a real change in bone mass occurs, whether enough change could be produced to be therapeutically useful.

Calcium. Availability of raw materials (principally calcium) is a further potential problem in the elderly. The lifelong dietary habits of the patient, typically characterized by a low calcium intake, are difficult to change. To further compound the problem, a major fraction of elderly women exhibit an impairment of calcium absorptive ability which is distinct from and in addition to the estrogen deprivation effect of menopause.[5,6] In some patients, the defect appears to be due to inadequate response of the renal mechanism for synthesis of $1,25(OH)_2D$ to exogenous parathyroid hormone (PTH); hence, increased calcium intakes may be required in the elderly to overcome what amounts to an absorptive block.

The importance of the rate of remodeling in changing bone mass has been established. A slow rate of remodeling limits bone loss; however, it also limits bone gain, even when providing therapy which might otherwise increase bone mass. Nutritional therapy of bone loss is an example of this problem. Calcium, once absorbed, acts to suppress PTH, which is the principal determinant of the quantity of bone remodeling in the normal adult. Hence, calcium therapy given for the purpose of repairing a deficiency of skeletal mass has the counterproductive effect of slowing bone remodeling. This makes the repair of a calcium deficit in an aging person qualitatively unlike the repair of other nutritional deficits (eg, iron-deficiency anemia, scurvy), in that repletion with the missing nutrient depresses the mechanism required for repair of the damage. This fact alone highlights the importance of preventing osteoporotic bone loss.

Miscellaneous Nutrients and Nutritional Interactions. Other nutrients have been implicated, rightly or wrongly, as contributing to bone loss. Protein is probably the most important of these. Inadequate protein intake creates a problem because bone matrix consists principally of protein; hence, protein is one of the raw materials required for skeletal integrity. Excessive protein intake can be a problem as well, and, for North Americans, presents more of a risk than does inadequate intake. Excess dietary proteins are, of course, metabolized and, in the process, the sulfur-containing amino acids are excreted as sulfuric acid.[7] This is associated with increased renal excretion of calcium, a kind of endogenous equivalent of the acid rain problem (in which limestone statues are gradually dissolved by being bathed in acid rain).

Excess dietary phosphorus has also been implicated, and in some animals it does appear to provoke bone loss. However, this does not appear to be the case in humans, and available evidence indicates no risk from this source.[7] In fact, if anything, the phosphorus associated with protein in most foods reduces the hypercalciuria otherwise associated with excess protein intake.

The status of other nutrients and nutrient interactions is less certain. Excess caffeine intake appears to exaggerate endogenous calcium loss and further increases the effective nutritional requirement for calcium.[7] Aluminum-containing antacids have a similar result because of their interference with calcium absorption. Finally, one should mention that sodium-restricted diets are, for all practical purposes, low-calcium diets as well, and thus, patients placed on such diets will need calcium supplements.

Role of Exercise in Rehabilitation. Although some patients with osteoporosis will not accept an exercise regimen, it must be pointed out that an aggressive muscle strengthening and retraining program can provide significant benefits for many of these patients. Primary emphasis should be given to strengthening the extensor muscles of the spine. In one sense, this retraining is analogous to the rehabilitation of poliomyelitis patients in whom remarkable results were sometimes achieved even in the face of extensive damage. The typical patient with osteoporosis is less severely handicapped than were many poliomyelitis victims, and the benefits of effective muscle strengthening and retraining can be considerable, both in terms of relief from pain and general well-being.

Other Forms of Treatment

In addition to diet and exercise, it is necessary to call attention to the status of other forms of therapy in connection with the treatment of osteoporosis. No regimen has yet been conclusively demonstrated to be efficacious in restoring lost bone. Estrogens have been used in the treatment of osteoporosis for many years, and the evidence indicates that their principal effect is to slow bone remodeling and to stabilize bone mass. Essentially no effective increase in bone mass occurs beyond that associated with the remodeling transient produced by treatment. Estrogens do not, therefore, fulfill the goal of increasing skeletal mass.

Fluoride, in varying doses, has been used to treat osteoporosis throughout the western world during the last decade. Unfortunately, very few adequately controlled studies have been done on the subject. Fluoride intoxication is associated with an exuberant overgrowth of bone. The rationale for the use of fluoride in the treatment of osteoporosis is based on the presumption that a controlled therapeutic level of fluoride can produce a useful increase in bone mass without undue toxicity. There appears to be little doubt that fluoride does indeed act as a potent stimulator of osteoblastic activity. The available evidence now indicates: 1) that trabecular bone mass increases; and 2) that spine fracture rate decreases, often dramatically.[8] There is some question as to whether cortical bone mass is affected, possibly even adversely, and there is great uncertainty about the effective dose level and the prevalence and management of untoward side effects, principally rheumatic and gastrointestinal complaints. Major studies are now underway to resolve several of these questions, and one can look forward to better answers in this area within the next few years.

Problem of Bone Mass and Fracture

In much of the research on osteoporosis, there is an assumption that decreased bone mass is the principal determinant of bone fragility. There is little doubt that bone mass is a major determinant of such fractures, and probably the most important such determinant; but it may not be the only one.

Clearly, people who have less bone are more likely to incur fractures than people who have more bone. The evidence for this conclusion is unequivocal. It is also true that some women with decreased bone mass somehow escape fracture. There are no good explanations for this phenomenon. Is this purely probabilistic? Or are other, unrecognized factors involved such as the superimposition of unrecognized osteomalacia; or the presence of ineffective remodeling, such that accumulated micro-fractures are not repaired; or finally something as simple as the propensity to fall? This is a nagging problem for which there are no satisfying answers. We need to look for such answers if we are ultimately to provide a satisfactory solution to the problem of osteoporosis.

Summary

Although diet and exercise play important roles in the maintenance of bone mass and in the prevention of osteoporosis, few studies have been done to demonstrate their role in formal therapy of the already existing disorder. There appear to be major practical impediments to their efficacy. First, exercise, while theoretically valuable, is very difficult to apply to a woman with a lifetime of relative inactivity, who is in pain and is to some degree disabled because of accumulated osteoporotic fractures. Secondly, nutritional therapy with calcium is limited in both the fact that elderly women absorb calcium less efficiently than do younger women, and also by the fact that without the stimulus provided by exercise, calcium can merely arrest further bone loss; it cannot, by itself, increase bone mass. These and other considerations highlight the importance of prevention as contrasted with treatment of osteoporosis.

References

1. Whedon GD: Interrelation of physical activity and nutrition on bone mass, in White PLW, Mondeika TM (eds): *Diet and Exercise: Synergism in Health Maintenance.* Chicago, American Medical Association, 1982, pp 99–112.

2. Parfitt AM: The integration of skeletal and mineral homeostasis, in DeLuca HF, Frost HM, Jee WSS, et al (eds): *Osteoporosis: Recent Advances in Pathogenesis and Treatment,* Baltimore, University Park Press, 1981, pp. 115–126.

3. Heaney RP, Recker RR, Saville PD: Menopausal changes in calcium balance performance. *J Lab Clin Med* 92:953–963, 1978.

4. Aloia JF, Cohn SH, Ostani JA, et al: Prevention of involutional bone loss by exercise. *Ann Int Med* 89:356–358, 1978

5. Gallagher JC, Riggs BL, Eisman J, et al: Intestinal calcium absorption and serum vitamin D metabolism in normal subjects and osteoporotic patients: effect of age and dietary calcium. *J Clin Invest* 64:729–736, 1979.

6. Slovik DM, Adams JS, Neer RM, et al: Deficient production of 1,25-Dihydroxyvitamin D in elderly osteoporotic patients. *N Engl J Med* 305:372–374, 1981.

7. Heaney RP, Recker RR: Effects of nitrogen, phosphorus, and caffeine on calcium balance in women *J Lab Clin Med,* In Press.

8. Riggs BL, Hodgson SF, Hoffman DL, et al: Treatment of primary osteoporosis with fluoride and calcium: clinical tolerance and fracture occurrence. *JAMA* 243:446–449, 1980.

Index

A

Abel, 148

Abramowitz, B.M. 148

Actin 51

Active Persons, see also Exercise; Sedentary Persons

    body fat   39, 44-45
    bone density   103-104
    diet   42-46
    energy intake   92
    exercise   93
    fat consumption   42-45
    hypertension   117-124
    lean body mass   75, 82
    and sedentary compared   39-42
    weight   39-40

Activity, see Exercise

Adenosime Triphosphate

    regeneration   52

Adipose Tissue, see also Body Fat; Obesity

    abdominal cells   93, 94
    exercise, effects   20
    hyperplastic   91, 93, 95
    lipolysis   56
    metabolic substrates   18-19
    sex differences   94, 96

Adolescents, see also Diabetes—Type I

    athletic training   33-34
    inactivity   28-32
    median caloric intake   30
    nutrition   29–34; iron   30,   32–33

Adult–Onset Diabetes, see Diabetes—Type II
Aging, see also Diabetes—Type II; Osteoporosis

    blood pressure levels   68-69
    bone loss—103-104, 107, 153-158
    hypertension   115
    physical activity   103-104

Alcohol   42, 44, 68

Allen, F.M.   69

Allison, T.G.   132

Aloia, J.F.   103, 104

Ambard, L.   69

Amery, A.   71

Amino Acids

    oxidation   54-59, 63; alamine   57-59; leucine   54-57 whole body metabolism   57-59

Androgens

    lean body mass, effects on   75-77, 80-81, 84-88

Anemia   33

Angina   128

Anorexia Nervosa   75-77, 82

Appetite Suppression   132

Arnold, J.S.   104

Aspen, A.J.   148

Astrand, P.O.   19, 22

Astronauts

    calcium loss   101-102, 105-106

Atherosclerosis   130, 138

    in diabetics   143–148

Athletic performance   15, 33-34

Atlee, C.   7

Avioli, L.V.   109

B

Bartley, M.H.   104

Bassett, C.A.L.   103

Bauer, W.   107

Beaujard, E.   69

Berg, A.   54

Beta–Endorphins 71

Bingert, A. 87

Blacks

    heart disease 9

Boddy, K. 83

Body Composition

    and exercise 44-45

Body Fat, see also Adipose Tissue; Obesity

    athletic performance 34
    energy imbalance 15
    exercise, effects 75, 82, 85, 91–95
    loss, and caloric intake 44-45
    of sedentary/active persons 39

Body Mass, see Lean Body Mass

Body Temperature

    regulation during exercise 16, 20-21

Body Weight, see also Obesity

    and activity 39-42
    androgen use 84-86
    exercise, effects 91-94; with diet 94; in severely obese 95
    and hypertension 70-72; in lean men 71
    and lean body mass 77, 81-86
    loss, glycemic control 145
    thermogenesis 93, 95-96

Bone Mass, see also Osteoporosis 99-110

    age-related loss 153-158
    aging 103-104, 107
    calcium intake 107-110; resorption 109, 155-158
    density 20, 103-104
    exercise, effects 103-104, 106, 109-110; and lean body mass 156
    fracture rates 108
    hypercalciuria 99-105
    inactivity, effects 99-102, 104, 109-110
    in menstruating women 103-108
    muscles, interrelationship 104, 106, 109
    osteomalacia 106
    osteoporosis 104, 107, 109
    remodeling 154-158
    rickets 106

Boileau, R.A.   83

Boyer,   72

Brodal, P.   19

Brown, C.H.   83, 86

Brozek, J.   86

Burmeister, W.   87

Buskirk, E.R.   17, 94

C

Calcium
> bone mass   107-109, 155-158
> in diet,   99-101, 104-110
> RDA   108, 155

Calloway, D.H.   54

Cancer
> lung   11

Carbohydrates
> exercise, effects   18-19; use of stored   55, 59
> fuel mix   51-52
> loading   55

Cathcart, E.P.   53

Carr, D.B.   71

Carter, J.E.L.   83

Celejowa, I.   60, 62

Cerny, F.   54

Children, see also Adolescents
> blood pressure levels   71, 72
> growth and exercise   50-51
> height/weight distributions   27-28
> poor nutrition   28-31

Cholesterol
> active persons   42
> coronary heart disease   42-45, 127, 130, 138
> in diabetics   147-149
> levels   7-9, 11

Cholesterol-Dietary   44-46

Cigarettes, see Smoking

Circulation

    exercise, effects   19-22

Coronary Heart Disease   7-12

    angina   128
    atherosclerosis   130, 138, 143-148
    cholesterol levels   42, 44-45
    diabetes   146-148
    diet   7-9
    exercise, benefits   7; effects   19-22, 39; risk   128-129; prevention   130; treatment programs   135-139
    hypertension   70-72; in lean men   71
    lipoprotein concentration   39
    mortality   7-12
    personality types   129, 134
    prevention   130-133
    risk factors   128-129
    sudden death   129

Consolazio, C. F.   60, 62, 83

Cornfield, J.   11

Creatinine Excretion   82

D

Davidson, J.K.   145

Davies, C.T.M.   87

Décombaz, J.   53-54

Diabetes   143-150

    diet   143-145
    hypertension   145, 147
    increased incidence   145
    vascular disease   143-148
    weight loss   145

Diabetes—Type I

    diet   143-144

Diabetes—Type II
  aerobic capacity 149
  coronary heart disease 146-148
  diet 144-145
  exercise, effects 146-148; training programs 148-150
  glucose homeostatis 146
  hypoglycemia 150
  insulin resistance 144-145
  target heart rate 150

Diet, see also Nutrition
  of active persons 42-45
  alcohol 42, 44, 68
  calcium 99-101, 104-110, 155-158
  carbohydrates 51-52
  diabetes 143-145; increased incidence of 145
  energy 94-95
  exercise, effects 42, 44-45
  fats 11, 42-45, 138
  fuel mix 51-52
  glycogen 52, 54
  hypertension 69-70
  iron 30, 32-33
  osteoporosis 155-158
  phosphates 106
  phosphorus 157
  plasma lipoproteins 44
  potassium 68, 70
  protein needs 60-63, 157
  sodium 67-70, 123
  vitamin D 106, 109

Drugs and Medications
  diuretics 70
  estrogen 157
  flouride 158
  glucosidase 145
  hypertension 11-12
  osteoporosis 157-158

Dohm, G.L. 55

Donaldson, H.H. 104

Doyle, F. 104

Durnin, J.V. 86

Dustan, H.R. 70

E

East, B.W. 87

Edholm, O.G. 31-32

Edwards, H.T. 93

Ehsani, A.A. 130

Ellis, K.J. 104

Emiola, L. 103

Energy
- expenditure 30-32; effect on exercise 91-93
- fuel mix 51-57
- imbalance and hypertension 115-124
- intake 28-30; effect on exercise 91-93
- muscle demand 59
- reserves 18-19
- stores of 51-52, 55, 59
- thermogenesis 93, 95-96

Epinephrine 20, 21, 93

Estrogen
- and osteoporosis 153, 155-157; medication 157

Evans County Study 71

Exercise, see also Active Persons; Athletic Performance; Sedentary Persons
- active persons, physical characteristics and diet 39-44
- aerobic 22-23, 52
- anabolic period 49, 60
- beta-endorphins 71
- body composition 44-45
- bones, effects on 103-104, 106, 109-110
- caloric intake 39-42, 44-45
- coronary heart disease, risk 128-129; prevention of 130; treatment programs 135-139
- diabetics, effects 146-148; training programs 148-150
- disease prevention 6-9
- duration 92, 134
- high-density lipoproteins, effects 130, 132
- hypertension, elevated during 71-72; effects 117-124
- lipid metabolism 39-46

    low-density lipoproteins, effects   130, 132
    motivation   17
    muscles, effects   49-51
    nitrogen excretion   52-54, 57, 63
    obesity   91-93
    osteoporosis   156-158
    plasma lipoprotein patterns   44-46
    protein, in diet   60-62
    regional effects   93, 96
    running   12, 17, 19
    sedentary persons   23
    serum cholesterol   12
    types and intensity   133
    urea production   52-54, 57
    walking   17, 23
    and weight   39-42

Exercise—Physiology   12-23

    adaptation   15-16
    metabolic substrates   18-19
    muscle contraction   16, 23
    regular, effects of   19-23
    temperature regulation   16, 20-21
    work measurement   16

F

Fahey, T.D.   83, 86

Fats

    fuel mix   51-52
    saturated   138

Fatty Acids

    exercise, effects   52, 55, 59

Felig, P.   57

Finch, C.A.   33

Framingham Study   70-71, 129, 134, 146

G

Gilliam, T.B.   31

Glucagon   19-22

Glucose Tolerance, see also Diabetes
    diet, effects 143-145
    exercise, effects 146, 149
    test 146, 149

Glycogen
    stored, use of 52, 54

Goldberg, A.L. 59

Goldman, R.F. 86

Gollnick, 25

Gontzea, I. 60-61

Gordon, T. 42

Grande, F. 21

Grover, J.A. 71

Growth Hormone 20-22

Guyton, A.C. 70

Gwinup, G. 91

H

Halberg, L. 32

Haralambie, G. 54

Hartung, G.H. 42

Heaney, R.P. 108-109

Heart
    exercise, effects 19-20, 22-23

Heart Disease, see Coronary Heart Disease

Hervey, G.R. 83-86

Hettinger, T. 16

High-Density Lipoproteins 20, 130, 132
    in active persons 42, 44-46
    coronary heart disease 42-45
    diabetes 147, 149
    diet 44-46

Homa, M. 60, 62

Hood, 148

Hypercalciuria 99, 105

Hyperglycemia 143-145

Hyperinsulimenia 145

Hypertension 147
> clinical studies 69-70
> coronary heart disease 11, 127-129, 138
> diabetes 145
> drug management 11-12
> epidemiology 68-69
> exercise, therapy 71; elevated during 72; effects 117-124
> experimental 70
> inactivity, effects 117-124
> in lean men 71
> and obesity 67, 70-71
> parental 117, 119-120
> sodium, effects 67-70, 123
> treatment 69-70, 71, 123

Hypertriglyceridemia 145, 147

Hypoglycemia
> in diabetics 150

Hypothalmus 21

I

Ingjer, F. 19

Insulin, see also Diabetes 21, 88, 93
> exercise, effects 146

Ireland, P. 109

Ireland-Boston Heart Study 7-9

Iron, see Vitamins and Minerals

Ischemic Heart Disease, see Coronary Heart Disease

J

James, F.W. 72

Jogging, see Running

Johnson, W.P. 71

Juvenile-Onset Diabetes, see Diabetes—Type I

K

Kasch, 72

Keen, H. 42

Kelly, J.M. 83

Kempner, W. 69

Keys, A. 86

Knuiman, J.T. 44

Knuttgen, H.G. 16, 22

Kramsch, D.M. 148

Krauss, R.M. 9

L

Lean Body Mass 75-88, 94
- androgen use 75-77, 80-81, 84-88
- exercise, effects 75-88, 156
- obesity 75-79, 82-83, 86-88
- pregnancy, during 75-76, 79, 85, 89
- sedentary/active persons compared 75, 82
- sexual development 84-85, 87
- in women 75-79, 82, 85, 87-88

Leaness, see Body Weight; Lean Body Mass

Lemon, P.W.R. 54-55

Leon, A.S. 83, 132

Leucine 54-59

Levy, A.M. 71

Ljunggren, H. 87

Liver
- metabolic demands 57, 59

Low-Density Lipoproteins 20, 130, 132
- active persons 42, 44-46
- and coronary heart disease 42-45
- diet 44-46

Lungs
    cancer   11
    exercise, effects   20, 22-23; oxygen consumption   52-57

M

Marable, N.L.   60

Maturity-Onset Diabetes, see Diabetes—Type II

Mayer, J.   92

Metabolism
    adipose tissue   18-19
    amino acids   54-59, 63
    calcium   99-101, 105-106
    carbohydrates   18-19
    exercise, effects, substrates   18-19; liver demands   57, 59
    fatty acids   19
    glycogen   19,20
    lipids   18
    lipoprotein lipase   19
    minerals   106
    proteins   51-57; in diet   60-63

Millward, D.J.   59

Mitochondria   59

Moody, D.L.   83

Morris, J.N.   42, 128-129, 134, 138, 146

Mullen, J.P.   54-55

Muscles
    adenosine triphospate regeneration   52
    alanine release   57-59
    amino acid oxidation   54-59, 63
    anabolicm   49, 60
    bone, interrelations   104, 106, 109
    contraction   16, 23
    energy reserves   18-19; demand   59
    exercise, effects   19-23, 49-51, 115
    fuel mix   51-57
    glycogen stores   52, 54
    metabolic substrates   18-19
    oxygen consumption   52-57

Myocardial Infarction, see Coronary Heart Disease

Myosin 51

N

Nitrogen

    caloric deprivation, loss during 75
    exercise, excretion during 52-54, 57, 63, 94, 95
    protein in diet 60-62
    sweat loss 54, 57, 61-62

Norepinephrine 20, 21, 93

Norgan, N.G. 86

Nutrition, see also Diet; Recommended Dietary Allowances

    bone mass, effects 106-110
    energy intake/expenditure 28-32
    essential nutrients 32-33
    lipid metabolism 39-46

O

Obesity, see also Adipose Tissue; Body Weight

    abdominal cells 93, 94
    caloric consumption 39, 42, 45
    children 27-28
    diabetics 143-145
    exercise, effects 91-93; regional effects 93, 96; and diet 94, 95; programs 95
    high risk persons 28
    hyperplasic adipose tissue 91, 93, 95
    hypertension 67, 70-71, 115-124
    lean body mass 75-79, 82-83, 86-88
    sex differences 94, 96

Odessey, R. 59

Oscai, L.B. 91-92

O'Shea, J.P. 103

Osteomalacia 106, 158

Osteoporosis 104, 107, 109, 153-158

    bone remodeling 154-158
    calcium 155-158
    estrogen 153, 155-157; as medication 157
    exercise program 156, 157, 158

Oxygen
  consumption during exercise 52-57

P

Paffenbarger, R.S. 128-129, 134, 138, 146-147

Page, L.B. 68-69

Parizkova, J. 82, 83

Personality Types 129, 134

Peterson, J. 76

Phillips, R.A. 3

Phillips. W.H. 83

Physical Activity, see Exercise

Plasma Lipoprotein
  and physical activity 39-42, 45
  diet, influence on 44-45

Poliomyelitis 100

Poortmans, J.R. 54

Pritikin Diet 44

Protein 106
  anabolic period 49, 60
  dietary needs 60-63
  growth and exercise 50-51
  metabolism, fuel mix 51-57; nitrogen excretion 52-54, 57, 63; oxidation 52-54, of amino acids 54-57

Pregnancy
  lean body mass 75-76, 79, 85, 88

Public Health
  coronary heart disease 7-12
  history 3
  mortality rates 7-12
  obesity 27
  physical activity 6-9
  Recommended Dietary Allowances 4-6, 17

Q

Qash'qai Study 68-69

R

Recommended Dietary Allowances 4-16, 17
     calcium, 108, 155

Reddan, W. 103-104

Refsum, H.E. 54

Reisin, E. 71

Rennie, M.J. 56

Respiration
     exercise, effects 20, 22-23; oxygen consumption 52-57

Rickets 106

Rodahl, K. 19, 22

Rosenman, R.H. 129

Running, see also Exercise 12, 17, 19
     and weight 39-40

S

Saltin, B. 149

Sasaki, N. 70

Saville, P.D. 104

Sedentary Persons, see also Active Persons; Exercise
     and active compared 39-42
     body fat 39
     calcium loss 99-102, 109-110
     caloric consumption 39-42
     exercise 93
     hypertension 117-124
     lean body mass 75, 82
     weight 39-42, 92

Seitchik, J. 88

Selvester, R. 130

Sherill, J.W.   69

Sinaki, M.   104

Skylab   101-102, 106

Smith, E.L.   103-104

Smoking

    cancer   11
    coronary heart disease   11-12, 127-130, 138, 147
    Surgeon Generals' report   11
    women   11

Sodium

    and hypertension   67-70, 123

Spady, D.W.   31

Spencer, H.   106

Stern, J.S.   95

Stroke   11-12

    exercise benefits   7

Strömme, S.B.   54

Sudden Death, see Coronary Heart Disease

Surgeon General, see U.S. Surgeon General

Sweat   16, 20-21

    loss during exercise   54, 57, 61-62

T

Ten State Nutritional Survey   27

Tanner, J.M.   82

Tarahumara Indians' Diet   44

Taylor, H.   21

Toss, L.   95

Triglyceride   94

U

U.S. Agriculture Department   4, 6, 12

    Daily Food Guide   4, 9, 12

U.S. Food and Nutrition Board   4-6, 9

U.S. Health, Education, and Welfare Department   9, 12

U.S. National Aeronautics and Space Administration   105

U.S. National Center for Health Statistics   27-28

U.S. National Institutes of Health   11

U.S. Surgeon General
 report on smoking   11

USDA Daily Food Guide   4, 9, 12

Urea
 exercise, effects of   52-54, 57, 63

V

Vagus Nerve
 heart rate, effect   20

Vitamins and Minerals
 iron   30, 32-33
 vitamin D   106, 109

Viteri, F.   50

W

Wahren, J.   57

Walking, see also Exercise   17, 23

Ward, P.   83, 86

Waterlow, J.C.   56

Weight, see Body Weight; Obesity

Wellness   17

West, K.M.   144

Western Collaborative Group
 study   129

Whedon, G.D.   155

Whyte, M.P.   104

Williams, B.T.   91-92

Wilmore, J.H.   83

Women, see also Estrogen; Pregnancy

    adolescents, inactivity   28-32
    anemia   33
    anorexia nervosa   75-77, 82
    athletes   33-34
    blood pressure levels   68
    calcium   108, 155
    caloric intake, active/inactive   40-41
    coronary heart disease   9, 129
    fat cell size   94, 96
    iron   30, 32-33
    lean body mass   75-79, 82, 85, 87-88
    osteoporosis   153, 155-158
    postmenopausal, bone formation   103, 108
    smoking habits   11

World Health Organization   3, 138

Y

Yano, K.   42